THE ULTIMATE GUIDE TO INTERMITTENT FASTING FOR WOMEN OVER 50

3 EFFECTIVE STRATEGIES TO LOSE WEIGHT, BALANCE HORMONES, AND REJUVENATE THE BODY AND THE MIND

FRANCIS J. LEIGH

FIRST THINGS FIRST

As you embark on your journey through this book, you will discover why it is important to break your fast with healthy, nutritious meals.

To give you some extra help, I would love to offer you a list of delicious recipes to support your quest to improve your well-being.

Just email the word 'recipes' to:
Francis@futurebalancenutrition.com

CONTENTS

INTRODUCTION

Have you ever reached a point in life when you felt like time was sprinting ahead, leaving you breathless in its wake? A moment when you looked in the mirror and wondered where the years had gone? Perhaps you've battled with changes in your body that seemed to pop up overnight, from stubborn weight gain to fluctuating energy levels. Or maybe you've navigated the uncharted waters of menopause, facing unpredictable symptoms that left you feeling like a passenger on an emotional roller coaster. You may have been told your body was letting you down because you are aging, or that hot flashes and mood swings are normal for your age.

You're not alone. Statistics show that countless women over 50 are grappling with these very challenges. According to recent studies, many women in this age group face a unique battle with their weight, a struggle that often feels like an uphill climb with no summit in sight (Gill et al., 2015).

But here's the thing: Turning 50 can be a pivotal moment when reflection and reevaluation become necessities. It's when you, like so many others, may find yourself seeking a path to rejuvenation and rekindling the sparks of life, rather than settling only for ways to slow your aging or solutions for your weight concerns.

I understand your journey because it's mine too. Despite leading a healthy life, when menopause hit, my health took a nosedive—gut problems, weight gain, emotional turbulence, brain fog, fatigue, you name it. But I refused to accept it as an inevitable part of aging. My body didn't feel like mine anymore, and I couldn't accept that the reason for this was that I was growing old! I wanted another answer—a practical response that would guide me to take action. So, that's what I sought.

I set off on a narrow road to turn back the clock and rediscover the vitality that I knew still resided within me. And I found the answer to my problems through intermittent fasting.

The Ultimate Guide to Intermittent Fasting for Women Over 50 is my gift to you. It's a transformative blueprint tailored specifically for you, a woman who's not content with simply accepting the status quo of aging. If you want to reshape your narrative for your future and to take back control of your health, let this be your guide to rewrite the story of your golden years.

In this guide, you'll discover a comprehensive understanding of intermittent fasting for women over 50. I won't just discuss the *how* of things but will comb through everything from *what* to *why*. I'll guide you as you explore the science behind intermittent fasting, exploring how it relates to the challenges of menopause and the post-50 landscape. You won't get a dizzying array of options here; instead, we'll focus on three effective intermittent fasting methods, each accompanied by clear, actionable steps.

You'll also find real-life success stories of women who have walked this path before you—women who have defied expectations and reclaimed their fitness. Although I must warn you that their stories aren't overnight miracles, the power of intermittent fasting is real because the change that follows is enough evidence.

I poured my dedication and research into crafting this guide to help other women who needlessly struggle. I've walked the path of trial and error that many undergo when trying to navigate aging and health. I also know what it's like to have days where I don't feel I have the energy to continue. That is why I'm not only excited but also passionate about leading you on this personal journey of change. Let's get started!

1

WOMAN IN HER PRIME—THE 50S AND BEYOND

Are you excited to uncover the secret to rejuvenating your body, losing unwanted weight, and balancing your hormones? Well, before we get there, let's discuss what happens to your body as you age—what is responsible for the changes that sometimes make your body feel strange.

I know about the fatigue and loss of self-esteem, the changes in mood and physical activity; you are not alone in this. A friend of mine—let's call her Trish—was always a lively soul and full of life. She enjoyed going for runs in the morning and swimming or biking with friends on weekends. But this all gradually changed when she was in her 50s because she started experiencing things she never dreamt would happen to her. She felt an unfamiliar twinge in her lower back, coupled with joint pain and sudden exhaustion.

This wasn't the Trish she knew. She felt like she lost the woman she once was; the invincible Trish, the one that could do anything. This also had a knock-on effect on her relationships as she started feeling less confident and avoiding friends. Not only was she a stranger to her body, but her mood was also different from how it used to be. One minute she could be happy and ready to take on the world. The next moment, she'd feel a little down, and her morale would be at an all-time low.

Many women just before and after hitting their 50s can relate to Trish's experience. A study found that 80% of women complained of different symptoms with different levels of severity during menopause (Grant et al., 2015).

This chapter focuses on helping you understand the major physical and emotional changes that we women go through when approaching and after turning 50 years of age. Knowing this will help you embrace the changes you're going through, and also equip you with the knowledge you need to make informed health decisions.

HORMONAL CHANGES

You've probably heard of hormones. Maybe you even have a tendency to blame your hormones when you are in a certain mood. But what precisely are they and why are they so important, especially for women in their 50s? In plain language, hormones are microscopic messengers that transport vital information from one place to another throughout your body. They play an important role in controlling a variety of body activities, ranging from metabolism to mood. These chemical messengers regulate your menstrual cycle, fertility, mood, and other bodily functions. They are responsible for the many stages of your life, including menarche, pregnancy, and menopause.

Overview of Menopause and Perimenopause

Perimenopause is a transitional phase that leads you to menopause, hence the name perimenopause. Think of it as a stage where your body begins to warn you to get ready for an incoming change, which typically begins in your 40s or earlier. During perimenopause, your hormone levels fluctuate, which may cause irregular periods and other symptoms, some of which we'll soon cover.

Menopause is the main event and is defined as a year of not having menstruation, without any pathological causes. While most women experience it in their early 50s, the timing varies widely.

Physical and Emotional Signs and Symptoms

The emotional and physical symptoms of perimenopause and menopause may be distinct from one another but may sometimes overlap.

Perimenopausal Signs and Symptoms

- **Irregular periods:** Your menstrual cycle may become as random as the weather, with lighter or heavier cycles and shifting dates.
- **Moodiness:** You may feel like your emotions are wildly going high and low, as if they are on a swing.
- **Sleep disturbances:** Night sweats and racing thoughts make it hard to get a good night's rest.
- **Changing sex drive:** You may experience changes in your libido as your desire to get intimate fluctuates, mostly being low.
- **Weight gain:** You may gain a lot of unwanted pounds, even without changing your usual diet.

Menopause Signs and Symptoms

- **Memory and concentration problems:** Sometimes, you may experience moments that feel like your mind went on a long vacation, and focusing on tasks becomes a little more difficult.
- **Hot flashes:** These are unexpected transient episodes of intense heat sensation you may experience, often accompanied by profuse sweating.
- **Mood swings:** It's common to have roller coaster emotions, with extreme highs and lows seemingly out of nowhere.

- **Night sweats:** You may struggle with episodes where you wake up drenched in sweat, and not because of a nightmare or any related event. Night sweats cause sleep disruption and may lead to exhaustion.

Your body may change differently from your friends in the same age group because of various factors, such as diet, physical activity, genetics, and more. What's the same for all of us, though, is that these changes are a normal part of the amazing experience of womanhood.

The Science Behind Perimenopause and Menopause

When you were young and transitioned to teenagehood, you noticed some changes, such as getting your period for the first time, your breasts becoming bigger, and your waist becoming more defined. This is because some hormones of interest called estrogen and progesterone had an important role in this. During puberty, your ovaries increase the production of both estrogen and progesterone, and this continues until you are in your 40s or 50s, when they eventually stop working. To help you understand the science more, let's look into the functions of estrogen and progesterone.

Estrogen

Think of estrogen as a protective agent with various functions in your body. It's in charge of making sure you release an egg every month and it also prepares your uterus for pregnancy.

Estrogen helps regulate your body temperature and keeps your bones strong. It also influences the production of serotonin, the "feel-good" hormone that helps stabilize your mood.

It's thanks to estrogen that your skin stays elastic and hydrated, which keeps it looking young. The hormone also helps maintain your hair health.

Estrogen keeps your blood vessels open and helps maintain your cholesterol levels in a healthy range, both of which are important for heart health.

Progesterone

The right progesterone levels improve your mood and help you feel calm. In pregnancy, progesterone helps maintain the uterine lining and provides a nurturing environment for a growing baby. The hormone also partners with estrogen to regulate your menstrual cycle. While estrogen prepares the stage, progesterone ensures a balanced and predictable cycle.

These two hormones work hand in hand to keep your body functioning harmoniously throughout your reproductive years. However, as you enter perimenopause and menopause, they become less synchronized, leading to the changes and symptoms we discussed earlier.

Now that you know the functions of these hormones, it can be easy to understand the perimenopausal and post-menopausal symptoms that Trish and other women out there experience.

As you enter perimenopause, your ovaries decide to take a break, and may not release eggs as regularly as before. The hormone production also becomes unbalanced, causing you to experience those unpredictable periods and mood swings.

In response to the drop in estrogen levels, your body's thermostat goes haywire and thinks you're overheating when you're not, and that's when you get sudden hot flashes.

When you reach menopause, your ovaries officially retire from their hormone-producing duties, and your body learns to adjust to this new normal, but it takes time.

Busting Myths About Perimenopause and Menopause

I used to think menopause started when a woman reached her 60s, so I didn't know what hit me when I found myself experiencing symptoms in my 40s. There are many misconceptions about menopause and the years leading up to it. In this section, I'll shed light on some of the more widespread myths so we can clear the air.

- **Hot flashes are the only symptom of menopause:** Despite hot flashes being a very common symptom presented in perimenopause and menopause, they are not the only symptoms that manifest during these phases of womanhood, and we have already covered more symptoms.
- **Only hormone replacement therapy (HRT) can treat menopause symptoms:** While HRT may help with some symptoms, it's not the only method available. Diet and exercise are just two examples of how a change in lifestyle can have a big impact during and prior to menopause.
- **There are no benefits to menopause:** You may have heard this a couple of times, but menopause liberates you from having monthly periods and using birth control.
- **All menopausal symptoms are severe:** It's not true that every woman goes through menopause with severe symptoms. Some people breeze through it with no problems at all, while others find it hard.
- **Weight gain is inevitable:** Weight gain can occur during perimenopause and menopause, but it's not a guarantee. Lifestyle choices, such as a balanced diet and regular exercise, play a substantial role in managing your weight, so we can't put all the blame on our hormones.

THE METABOLIC SLOWDOWN

You may wonder why you have put on some extra pounds without even changing the diet you have been following for the past decade or more. This was one of my problems, too—I couldn't understand why I was gaining extra weight even though I kept the same diet. It bothered me until I discovered how metabolism changes as we age.

You probably hear this word often, but metabolism refers to the chemical process that helps create energy in your body. When you consume food and liquids, your body converts that into energy to power all bodily functions, from breathing to marathon running, and even cellular processes.

Basal Metabolic Rate (BMR)

Another concept you need to be familiar with is the basal metabolic rate. It's the energy your body uses to keep the body running at rest while maintaining basic physiological functions. Your BMR accounts for about 70% of the energy you burn daily. Everyone's basal metabolic rate is different, and it depends on several factors which are listed below:

- **Body composition:** Your body composition is one of the most important factors influencing BMR. At rest, muscle burns more calories than fat. As a result, if two people are the same weight, but have different muscle-to-fat ratios, their BMRs are different.

- **Age:** Our BMR naturally decreases as we age, and we'll soon cover this.
- **Gender:** The BMRs of men and women differ in that men have more muscle mass than women (Schorr et al., 2018), implying a higher BMR.
- **Genetics:** Your genes have an impact on your BMR as some people are born with a fast metabolism, while others are born with a slow metabolism. This is why you can notice metabolic differences even among family members.
- **Hormones:** The thyroid hormone is important for moderating metabolic processes, so if someone has a thyroid problem, the condition also affects their BMR. As a result, thyroid disorders result in significant metabolic changes.
- **Functions:** Exercising does more than just burn calories; it also affects your BMR. Regular exercise, particularly strength training, may boost your BMR by preserving and increasing muscle mass.

Why Metabolism Slows Down During Perimenopause and at Menopause

The slowdown of metabolism during menopause is influenced by numerous physiological changes, as listed below.

- **Estrogen reduction:** The decrease in estrogen production during menopause and perimenopause also affects your metabolism, changing things like how much energy is expended, distributed fat, and body weight. Lower estrogen levels make your body less effective at using glucose as fuel, which may result in insulin resistance. This may lead to weight gain and a lessened capacity to utilize food calories effectively.
- **Loss of muscle mass:** As we get older, we naturally lose muscle mass. Your BMR declines as you lose muscle, which also slows down metabolism.
- **Changes in fat distribution:** Estrogen affects the location of fat storage in your body. Lower estrogen levels are linked to an increased risk of health problems and metabolic changes, as well as a propensity to store more fat in the abdominal region.
- **A reduction in physical activity:** Due to symptoms such as joint pain and fatigue, you may

feel like reducing your physical activity levels during menopause. However, reduced physical activity leads to muscle loss and further contributes to a slower metabolism.

- **Changes in appetite control:** The hormone estrogen also plays a role in regulating your appetite, but during menopause, you may experience changes in hunger and satiety cues. This shift may have an effect on your total calorie intake and, in turn, your metabolism.

Impact of Slow Metabolism on Weight

- **Weight gain:** One of the most noticeable effects of a slower metabolism during menopause is an increased propensity for weight gain, particularly around the abdominal area. This change in fat distribution is often frustrating and may lead to concerns about body image.
- **Challenges in weight management:** It often becomes more challenging to maintain or lose weight during and after menopause. The combination of hormonal changes, decreased muscle mass, and metabolic shifts make it easier to gain weight and more difficult to shed those extra pounds.
- **Risk of obesity:** The unintentional weight gain may lead to obesity if it goes unmanaged. Obesity is associated with various health risks, including

cardiovascular disease, diabetes, and certain
cancers (Panuganti et al., 2022), making it crucial
to address weight concerns during menopause.

Regarding your general well-being, the metabolic slow-down also interferes with bone health, insulin resistance, and cardiovascular health. The metabolic slowdown may affect bone density, potentially leading to osteoporosis. This condition makes bones fragile and more susceptible to fractures. Changes in metabolism may also influence cholesterol levels and increase the risk of heart disease. The decrease in estrogen levels may contribute to insulin resistance, a condition where cells don't respond well to insulin. This may lead to higher blood sugar levels and an increased risk of type 2 diabetes. Weight gain and hormonal changes may put additional stress on joints, potentially leading to joint pain or exacerbating conditions like osteoarthritis.

AGE-RELATED CONCERNS

It's no secret that aging has its own concerns, but not all of them are common knowledge. In this section, I'll share some concerns you may have as you age.

Bone Density

Bones are an integral part of the body, but as we age and go through menopause, our bone density changes. Bone density matters because it ensures that your bones remain strong and able to withstand the force placed upon them. Good bone density also facilitates fracture prevention, especially in high-stress areas, such as the hip, spine, and wrist. Reduced bone density makes the bones fragile, leaving them more prone to breakage. Strong bones are also essential for maintaining mobility and independence as you age. They allow you to move, walk, and perform daily activities with confidence.

During menopause, when estrogen levels decline, there's a heightened risk of decreased bone density, a condition known as osteoporosis. This is because estrogen promotes the activity of bone-forming cells called osteoblasts to help maintain bone density by building new bone tissue. Estrogen also inhibits bone-resorbing cells called osteoclasts. However, as you reach menopause and estrogen levels decline, the delicate balance between bone formation and resorption is disrupted. Bone resorption may outpace bone formation, leading to a gradual decrease in bone density.

The most immediate risk of decreased bone density is an increased susceptibility to fractures, particularly in the hip, spine, and wrist. These fractures can be debilitating and impact your quality of life. Weakened bones in the spine may also lead to a stooped posture and a noticeable reduction in height. Fragile bones may cause chronic pain and limit your mobility, making daily activities challenging. Severe bone density loss may result in a loss of independence and increased reliance on others for daily tasks.

Muscle Mass

Age-related natural muscle loss is a normal occurrence, and this gradual loss of muscle tissue is referred to as sarcopenia.

After the age of 30, muscle mass typically declines by 3–8% per decade. After the age of 60, though, the rate of decline increases even more (Volpi et al., 2004).

The decline in muscle mass, strength, and function that comes with aging is a major cause of disability in the elderly. It may result in a loss of mobility, an increase in frailty, and a higher risk of fractures and falls.

In addition, as your body becomes less effective at using calories from food, a lower BMR makes it easy to put on weight, possibly resulting in obesity and associated health problems. Keep in mind that as your muscle mass declines, your body burns less calories at rest, which lowers your BMR.

Other Age-Related Concerns

As you get older, you may encounter changes in your vision. You may struggle with conditions such as cataracts, age-related macular degeneration, and presbyopia (difficulty focusing on close objects). Joint health is another concern that arises with age. As you grow older, maintaining joint health becomes more critical for comfort and mobility.

Health problems such as heart disease and hypertension are more likely to develop the older you get. Your quality of life could be impacted if they are not controlled. Another concern that may arise with age is a decline in cognitive function, which affects areas such as your memory and ability to solve problems.

EMOTIONAL WELL-BEING: THE ROLE OF HORMONES AND LIFE TRANSITIONS

For many women, life after 50 can feel like a roller coaster ride of shifting emotions, and there's an understandable reason behind that. I remember the days I would wake up feeling on top of the world, full of energy, and ready to conquer whatever challenges would come my way. The next day, though, I would find myself drowning in sorrow with unexplained mood swings. I didn't know what was happening to me, and sometimes I thought it was just the loneliness from my children leaving home to go live independently. Little did I know other women in their 50s and beyond were already going through similar situations!

When Trish came to me complaining about how her moods were becoming unstable, I looked at her and smiled. She thought something was wrong with her, but I told her there was an explanation behind it all.

I know the stage of life you are in can make you unhappy on some days, but I assure you there is a fix for that. I'll soon share the secrets of thriving after 50, but first, let's look into why you may experience emotional instability during that phase.

The Link Between Estrogen and Serotonin

The levels of estrogen in your body have a huge role to play in mood regulation. Among those numerous functions, estrogen is involved in controlling mood. However, the reduced levels of estrogen during and after menopause impact the hormone serotonin, which functions as a neurotransmitter essential for controlling mood, emotions, and some physiological processes. As I said earlier, it's sometimes called the feel-good hormone because of its connection to positive emotions such as happiness. When serotonin levels are low or its receptors aren't functioning optimally, you may experience feelings of sadness, hopelessness, and a general decrease in mood.

Serotonin is produced and works better in the brain when estrogen levels are constant. In turn, serotonin aids in controlling mood, anxiety, and even sleep habits. Simply put, you're more likely to feel emotionally stable and happy when your estrogen levels are balanced.

Empty Nest Syndrome

When children move out of the house to live independently, parents may suffer from empty nest syndrome, which is characterized by feelings of sadness, loss, and loneliness. The condition can be particularly challenging because you dedicated a significant portion of your life to raising your children, so it's natural to struggle with finding a new sense of purpose and identity without them.

I know the feeling because I have been there. I became a single mother of two in my 20s, so taking care of my children and providing for them became part of my identity. But time moves fast and my little bundles of joy became all grown up and decided to move out and explore their lives on their own. Who am I to stop them? After all, we raise children in hopes that they will become independent. Still, it hit me hard. How was I supposed to live without their bustling laughs, endless conversations, and their comforting presence? I was already failing to cope without my children, but coupling that change with menopause sent my life spiraling out of control. Now, I take comfort in knowing I'm not the only one because research shows that depression is common among empty nesters (Yao et al., 2019).

Why People Get Empty Nest Syndrome

- **Children leaving home:** The most obvious cause is when children move away from home, whether it's for school, a job, or to start their own families.
- **Identity shift:** For many mothers, being a parent plays a vital part in who they are. By virtue of being a mother, you may struggle with issues of identity and purpose when your children depart.
- **Role shifts:** As parenting responsibilities and daily routines change, there is a corresponding shift in roles. You may find yourself suddenly having more free time and grieving the loss of your previous position as a full-time parent.

The Emotional Impact

Studies found that 73.3% of empty nesters had signs of depression. 63.4% of them had mild depression, while 9.9% had depression that was moderate to serious (Song et al., 2023).

The emotional effects of empty nest syndrome vary from person to person, but they often include the following:

- **Depression and grief:** Many mothers experience a deep sense of loss when their children leave home. The empty house can serve as a constant reminder of their absence, leading to feelings of sadness and even grief.
- **Loneliness:** The sudden reduction in social interactions in the house may cause a sense of isolation and loneliness.
- **Identity crisis:** You may grapple with questions about your identity and purpose. You may even find yourself wondering who you are outside of your role as a parent.
- **Anxiety and uncertainty:** Not knowing what the future holds can lead to anxiety. You may worry about your children's well-being and whether you have adequately prepared them for the challenges they will face in the outside world.
- **Mixed emotions:** It's important to note that empty nest syndrome isn't solely characterized by negative emotions. Some mothers experience a mix of emotions, including pride in their children's independence and excitement about the possibilities that lie ahead.

Coping With Empty Nest Syndrome

I personally struggled with this time in my life, as I mentioned previously. Eventually, though, I was able to use the opportunity and the newfound free time to reinvent myself. You, too, can learn new ways to improve both yourself and your life.

Positivity about oneself is the first step in coping with empty nest syndrome. Even if you have other commitments to handle, try putting self-care and self-discovery at the top of your list. Explore new skills or interests, or go back to old ones that you may have put on hold while you were raising kids. Use the first hour of the day for yourself and fill your cup first—something you have unlikely done for a very long time!

Another effective way to overcome empty nest syndrome is communication. Keep in touch through calls, texts, or visits to help ease the pain of being apart from your family. You may also expand your circle by building relationships with other moms going through menopause. Some exciting options for a start include getting back in touch with old friends, joining clubs, or doing something for the community.

If your feelings become overwhelming or cause you a lot of pain, you might also want to try therapy or counseling.

KEY TAKEAWAYS

Here are the key takeaway points from what we discussed in this chapter.

Hormonal changes:

- Menopause and perimenopause are natural phases in your life, characterized by significant hormonal shifts.
- Mood swings, hot flashes, and irregular periods are some of the physical and mental manifestations that can result from hormonal changes.
- In order to successfully navigate this phase, it's crucial for you to learn the science underlying these hormonal changes.

The metabolic slowdown:

- Metabolism refers to the body's processes for converting food into energy. The basal metabolic rate (BMR) is a significant determinant of metabolic speed and is subjected to changes throughout time.
- BMR naturally declines with age, impacting the rate at which your body burns calories at rest.
- This slowdown contributes to weight gain and other age-related health concerns.

Age-related concerns:

- Apart from metabolism slowing down, other age-related concerns include changes to bone density, muscle mass, vision, joint health, cardiovascular health, and cognitive function.
- These aspects of health are vital for your general well-being, and their decline is a natural part of aging.

Emotional well-being:

- Hormonal changes, particularly the connection between estrogen and serotonin, may influence your emotional well-being.
- As estrogen levels decline, it can disrupt the balance of serotonin in your brain, leading to mood swings and emotional fluctuations.

Empty nest syndrome:

- Empty nest syndrome is a phase that many mothers experience when their children leave home to pursue independence, further their education, work away from home, or other similar reasons.
- The emotional impact includes sadness, loneliness, identity shifts, and even anxiety.

- Coping strategies involve maintaining communication with children, prioritizing self-care, fostering social connections, and seeking professional help if the condition becomes difficult to manage.

Although aging is a natural part of life, how we handle our health and well-being also influences how we age. I'll discuss the advantages of intermittent fasting and how it benefited many women over 50, including myself, in the following chapter. It has the potential to solve the menopausal challenges we've covered, bringing about hormonal balance, increased vitality, and a better awareness of our bodies. I certainly experienced the first signs of improvement in just a few days. Read on to discover intermittent fasting demystified!

2

THE BASICS OF INTERMITTENT FASTING

A study showed that from 2013 to 2016, about 49.1% of adults in the US alone tried to lose weight, with women having a higher percentage of 56.4% than men at 41.7% (Centers for Disease Control and Prevention, 2018). On a global scale, 52% of adults worldwide are attempting to lose weight (Mark, 2022).

After turning 50, losing weight can be especially challenging, given the unique physiological changes we tend to experience. However, intermittent fasting has demonstrated itself as the light at the end of the tunnel we have been looking for. Today, millions of people all around the world are experimenting with intermittent fasting as a dietary plan for shedding pounds while improving their health overall. According to studies, intermittent fasting can significantly improve your weight management, heart health, mental clarity, and emotional health (Kandola, 2023).

THE BASICS OF INTERMITTENT FASTING

Remember my friend Trish from the first chapter? The problems she was going through got resolved after I introduced her to intermittent fasting. I understand your struggles the same way I related to hers because I went through it too. In this chapter, we'll look into the principles of intermittent fasting and explore why it's turning into the go-to method for women, especially after 50 years of age.

Cycling between times of fasting and eating is a key component of the intermittent fasting dietary strategy. It's not a specific diet, but an eating pattern that dictates when you should eat, rather than what you should eat.

The use of intermittent fasting for improving health is not a new concept—it has a long history. Fasting was a common practice among ancient civilizations like the Greeks and Romans for a variety of reasons, from religious rites to health advantages. Research proves that fasting was seen as a way to cleanse the body and achieve a higher level of spiritual enlightenment while promoting self-discipline and strengthening one's mental and physical resilience (Visioli et al., 2022).

Our hunter-gatherer ancestors also experienced periods of feast and famine due to the unpredictability of food availability. This evolutionary history may have shaped our ability to adapt to periods of food scarcity. It's an essential part of the narrative when discussing the benefits of intermittent fasting, as it reflects how our bodies are designed to handle variations in food intake.

Even though different religions still maintained fasting, in more recent history, intermittent fasting gained attention in the 20th century through scientific research and studies. One notable study conducted in the 1940s found that rats subjected to intermittent fasting lived longer and experienced fewer age-related diseases (Stipp, 2013). This sparked further interest and exploration into the potential health benefits of fasting.

The Difference Between Calorie-Based and Intermittent Fasting

Learning the major differences between intermittent fasting and other diets is important for you to understand intermittent fasting as a revolutionary lifestyle choice, rather than as simply another diet.

Here are some ways in which intermittent fasting varies from other eating regimens:

- **Shift in focus:** Food and calorie intake are often the focus of many diets. On the other hand, intermittent fasting largely concentrates on when you eat. Putting a greater emphasis on meal timing rather than stringent dietary restrictions redefines your relationship with food.
- **Sustainability:** Diets are usually associated with short-term plans to reach certain goals, such as weight loss. However, intermittent fasting is made to last for a long time instead of providing a "quick fix" way to lose weight.
- **Flexibility:** A lot of diets impose strict guidelines and restrictions on what dieters eat. Flexible and adaptable eating conditions make intermittent fasting an exciting journey. It doesn't label entire food categories or designate all your favorite foods as forbidden. Instead, it offers a framework that you may use to make wiser decisions regarding your eating habits.
- **Holistic well-being:** Intermittent fasting offers a wider range of health advantages than common diets that typically concentrate only on weight loss. It's important to promote general well-being, including hormonal balance, a faster metabolism, and even potential long life, in addition to weight loss.

- **Mindful eating:** The practice of intermittent fasting encourages conscious eating. You can establish a stronger connection with your body's hunger and satiety cues by being aware of when you eat and how your body reacts to food.
- **Lifestyle integration:** Intermittent fasting is a lifestyle you can easily incorporate into routine activities. It doesn't call for specialty foods or complex meal planning. Instead, it fits in with your daily routines, increasing the chances of long-term sustainability.

THE SCIENCE BEHIND FASTING

Instead of just taking my word for it, you may be curious to discover the science behind intermittent fasting.

Intermittent fasting is like giving your digestive system a break so your body can focus on other vital functions. You separate your day into two parts: the times when you eat and the times when you don't. For instance, you could only eat from 12 p.m. to 8 p.m., then fast the rest of the time.

When you eat, your body breaks down the food into energy and stores excess energy in the form of glycogen in your liver and muscles, and as fat in adipose tissue. In times of fasting, especially during prolonged periods, your body begins to tap into these stored energy reserves to keep other bodily functions running.

When you fast, your hormones change in important ways that are key to how well it works. One of the main hormones affected by fasting is insulin, a hormone produced from the pancreas, which helps cells take in and store glucose. Eating raises your blood sugar, and that triggers your body to release insulin. During a fast, your insulin levels decrease, making it easier for your body to use stored fat as energy.

Phases of Fasting

The phase your body enters just after you have a meal is called the fed state. During this time, your digestive system actively breaks down the food you ate into various nutrients, such as carbohydrates and proteins. Your body uses glucose from carbohydrates as its primary energy source and stores any excess glucose that is not immediately used. The energy is either stored as glycogen in the liver and muscles or converted to fat and stored for later use. Insulin plays an important role in the nutritional state as it helps move glucose out of your bloodstream and into the cells, where it can be used for energy or stored.

Early Fasting State

As you move into the early fasting state, typically a few hours after your last meal, your body's glucose levels begin to drop. At this point, insulin levels decrease, allowing your body to shift gears metabolically. Another hormone called glucagon comes into play here. This hormone enables your body to break down glycogen to glucose for energy in a process called glycogenolysis. Remember, glycogen is the stored form of glucose, and it's readily accessible for quick energy. This phase can last for several hours, depending on factors such as your last meal's composition and your activity level.

The early fasting state is marked by a decline in blood sugar levels and a shift toward using glycogen as the primary energy source. Your body begins to prepare for a more extended period of fasting while transitioning from the fed state.

The Fasting State

As glycogen stores become depleted, your body starts to rely more on stored fat for energy. This sets the stage for further metabolic shifts as you progress into longer fasting periods. Insulin levels remain low during the fasting state, making your body access and break down fat stores. This process is known as lipolysis. As fat molecules break down, they release energy in the form of fatty acids and glycerol, which your cells then use for fuel.

Ketone production also increases during the fasting state. Ketones are molecules produced when fat breaks down, and they serve as an alternative fuel source for your brain and muscles. This shift to using fat and ketones for energy is a key feature of the fasting state and is often associated with benefits such as weight loss, improved mental clarity, and improved metabolic health.

Long-Term Fasting State

You enter the starvation state after going without food for a prolonged length of time, usually more than 48 hours. Your body now relies on fat as its main energy source and gradually adjusts to using fat reserves. This shift produces high levels of ketones in a process called ketosis.

Even though your body can adapt to using fat for energy, it still needs some glucose. Using non-carbohydrate sources including amino acids and glycerol, your body can produce some glucose through a process known as gluconeogenesis.

The long-term fasting state is characterized by significantly decreased hunger and a significant metabolic shift in favor of utilizing fat reserves. It causes major weight loss in addition to providing other metabolic benefits. However, because of the risks involved and the fact that it may not be suitable for everyone, I recommend getting a medical opinion from a credible health professional before starting prolonged fasting.

THE MYRIAD BENEFITS OF INTERMITTENT FASTING

The physical and emotional transformations Trish went through left her questioning her identity, just like a lot of other women in their 50s. One day, during our discussions about health and well-being, I introduced Trish to the concept of intermittent fasting. I explained how this lifestyle could potentially provide her with the tools she needed to regain control over her body, balance her hormones, and rejuvenate her spirit. I was honest with her and told her it's not a magic pill, but a path to empowerment through mindful eating and structured fasting periods.

Trish was intrigued and decided to give intermittent fasting a try. I could see the determination in her eyes as we worked together to create a fasting schedule that suited her lifestyle and preferences. It was a gradual process, but her open heart allowed her body to adapt and her mindset to shift.

As with every new approach, the initial stages had their challenges. Trish complained about hunger pangs and she had moments of doubt, but she persevered. She drew strength from the knowledge that this journey was about more than just losing weight or addressing physical symptoms. I had told her it would give her control over her life and improve how she viewed herself.

After some months, Trish began to reap the benefits of her commitment. She told me her energy levels were becoming more stable, and I also noticed her mood swings started to mellow. The extra weight she had carried for years began to gradually melt away, returning the confident woman I knew.

Apart from the physical changes Trish was happy about, anyone could feel the sense of empowerment that radiated from her every word and action. She shared with me that intermittent fasting made her feel more in control of her body and life than ever before.

Trish's story shows the transformative power of intermittent fasting, especially for women after menopause. Her journey is a reminder that you have the capacity to shape your own destiny and embrace the empowered woman within. Discover some benefits of this eating approach below.

Insulin Sensitivity

As we discussed earlier, insulin's main job is to help glucose move from the bloodstream into cells, where it can be used for energy or stored as glycogen or fat. However, eating a lot of high-carbohydrate meals and snacks causes your blood sugar to rise and fall all the time, which increases your insulin levels. Over time, this may make the body's cells less sensitive to the effects of insulin, giving rise to a new problem called insulin resistance. Insulin resistance is a sign of type 2 diabetes and is linked to a number of health problems, such as weight gain and heart disease.

This is where intermittent fasting swoops in to set you back on the right track. Fasting periods, especially those that extend for several hours, lead to a reduction in insulin levels. This is because your body won't need to continually manage incoming glucose from food when you eat after several hours.

As your insulin levels decrease during fasting, cells become more receptive to the hormone's effects. This increased sensitivity means that when the body finally produces insulin, the hormone can transport glucose into cells more efficiently.

Improved insulin sensitivity also helps maintain stable blood sugar levels throughout the day, and that reduces your risk of having energy crashes and sugar cravings. It also lowers the likelihood of sudden spikes and crashes in insulin, which may contribute to weight gain.

The ability of intermittent fasting to enhance insulin sensitivity contributes to more efficient fat burning and may aid in weight loss or weight maintenance. Visceral fat, which is particularly hazardous to health, may also be reduced with intermittent fasting.

Improved insulin sensitivity lowers your risk of having type 2 diabetes and metabolic syndrome. It also plays a role in improving cardiovascular health, as it contributes to better blood vessel function and reduced inflammation.

Metabolism and Fat Loss

By now, you already know that intermittent fasting leads to weight loss by making the body use stored fat as an energy source during fasting periods. More importantly, this approach tends to target fat while preserving muscle, which is a positive outcome that many people fail to attain when following other common diets.

In addition, fasting triggers a cascade of hormonal changes, some of which have a positive impact on your metabolism. Another advantage is that the increase in growth hormone levels during fasting supports muscle growth and repair. With this, it becomes easier for you to maintain lean muscle mass, which is crucial for a healthy metabolism because muscle burns more calories at rest than fat. If you remember, muscle mass plays a crucial role in restoring your metabolism, and because women tend to lose more muscle with age, this is good news.

Autophagy

I know the word "autophagy" may sound strange to many, but I'll soon break it down and explain how it relates to intermittent fasting. It's a Greek word that means "self-eating" (De Rechter et al., 2015).

Picture your cells as houses; over time, broken parts and even dangerous invaders like viruses and bacteria build up inside. Autophagy is the process that finds and gets rid of this cellular trash, reusing what it can. It's a carefully controlled process that happens inside your cells and works like a cleaning crew.

Here is why it's important for cell health:

- **Cellular rejuvenation:** Autophagy helps cells get new life by getting rid of old or broken parts. This ensures that your cells work at their best and can do various activities well.
- **Disease prevention:** A properly functioning autophagy system is associated with a reduced risk of various diseases including Alzheimer's and Parkinson's and other neurodegenerative conditions, as well as some cancers. The process helps protect your cells from dysfunction or cancer by eliminating harmful proteins and removing damaged cell structures.
- **Immune contribution:** Autophagy also plays a role in the immune system. It helps destroy aggressive bacteria and viruses and protects your body against infection.

Fasting, especially during prolonged periods, triggers autophagy as your body looks for alternative sources of energy when you're not consuming food. When the primary energy source, glucose, is scarce, your body starts breaking down cellular components, including damaged ones, for energy.

Intermittent fasting, with its cycles of eating and fasting, is a natural way to stimulate autophagy. Giving your body extended breaks between meals provides it with the opportunity to engage in this cellular cleanup process regularly.

Inflammation

Your body naturally experiences inflammation as a reaction to injury or illness, but when it persists for an extended period, it may lead to a variety of health problems. Again, intermittent fasting comes in as an effective ally in the struggle against chronic inflammation.

Here is how it helps:

- **Decreases inflammatory markers:** Intermittent fasting has been linked to a drop in C-reactive protein (CRP) and interleukin-6 (IL-6), two of the body's inflammatory markers (Mulas et al., 2023). Some medical conditions, such as heart disease, diabetes, and some autoimmune diseases, are linked to these markers. Intermittent fasting helps bring down the overall amount of inflammation by lowering the markers.
- **Balanced blood sugar:** We have already discussed how intermittent fasting improves insulin sensitivity and stabilizes your blood sugar. This stabilizes blood sugar levels and promotes better metabolic health and less inflammation.
- **Enhanced antioxidant defense:** Studies have shown that fasting may trigger an increase in

antioxidant defenses in the body (Gîlcă et al., 2003). Antioxidants help combat oxidative stress, which is a major contributor to inflammation. This means you can use intermittent fasting to reduce inflammation caused by free radicals.

- **Weight management:** Excess body fat is associated with increased inflammation, but intermittent fasting supports weight loss and the reduction of visceral fat. As you shed excess weight, you're likely to notice a decrease in inflammation.

Intermittent fasting works as a natural anti-inflammatory by lowering inflammatory markers, helping cells clean up, balancing blood sugar, boosting defenses, assisting in weight regulation, and improving metabolic health as a whole.

Reducing the Chances of Age-Related Diseases

Research suggests that intermittent fasting may extend lifespan by improving metabolic health and reducing the risk of age-related diseases (Stipp, 2013). Who wouldn't want all these benefits? Here are more advantages of intermittent fasting:

- **Coronary heart disease:** You can address the risk factors for coronary heart disease by aiming for reduced weight loss, lower blood pressure, and improved insulin sensitivity which are all results of intermittent fasting.

- **Rheumatoid arthritis:** As discussed, intermittent fasting helps reduce chronic inflammation, a key driver of autoimmune diseases such as rheumatoid arthritis. Lowering inflammation gives intermittent fasting its potential to alleviate symptoms and improve the quality of life for individuals with autoimmune conditions.

- **Brain health:** Neuronal growth and maintenance are supported by the protein brain-derived neurotrophic factor (BDNF), which is produced in response to fasting. It also promotes the development of new brain cells and enhances cognitive function. This contributes to better brain health and may reduce your risk of developing neurodegenerative diseases, such as Alzheimer's and Parkinson's.

- **Gut health:** Your gut flora can be kept in a balanced state by intermittent fasting. A diverse and balanced microbiome promotes better digestive health, helps reduce inflammation, and contributes to an improved immune function. All these benefits may protect you against gut-related conditions while supporting your overall wellness.

Other Holistic Benefits

- **Simpler eating patterns:** Intermittent fasting makes meal planning and eating schedules simpler. This simplicity may lead to a more thoughtful and balanced approach to food by reducing the desire to constantly snack or develop bad eating habits.
- **Taking back control of your body:** Menopause might occasionally make you feel as though you no longer have control over your body. You could feel as though your body is betraying you as a result of hot flashes, mood swings, and weight changes. Intermittent fasting introduces a sense of agency. You actively choose when and how you eat, establishing a pattern that supports your tastes and goals. Having this control over your food habits can be powerful.
- **Increased energy and vitality:** You can experience an increase in energy and vitality as a result of intermittent fasting's ability to control blood sugar levels and enhance energy utilization. This increase in physical vitality may result in more excitement and optimism in your day-to-day activities.
- **Sense of accomplishment:** A feeling of accomplishment can come from successfully implementing intermittent fasting into your way of life. It's a commitment to your health, and you'll

probably feel more confident and self-assured when you see good improvements like weight loss, improved metabolic markers, and higher energy.

- **Sense of community:** Online or in-person supportive communities are common for menopausal women who are interested in intermittent fasting. Sharing experiences, struggles, and accomplishments with other women like you helps lessen feelings of loneliness by fostering a sense of community and emotional support.

THE SCIENCE OF HUNGER: NAVIGATING YOUR BODY'S SIGNALS DURING FASTING

Now that we have discussed how intermittent fasting works, and you have read about its benefits, you may feel ready to start. But, there is one other thing we need to look at—hunger. We all have those times when we just want to chew something; not because we're hungry, but maybe because we're bored, anxious, or simply curious! This raises the question: How do you recognize true hunger while fasting?

Let's start by defining hunger, which is a basic physiological response that signals your body's need for food. You may feel this in the form of a physical sensation such as your stomach rumbling.

Hormones, neural messages, and psychological factors all work together to control hunger. Ghrelin and leptin are the main hormones that control hunger. Ghrelin is often called the "hunger hormone" because it's responsible for making you hungry. Its levels usually increase right before meals, telling your body it's time to eat. Leptin, the "satiety hormone," tells your brain when you have eaten enough. The hormone is made by fat cells and its levels rise after a meal to make you feel full and stop you from eating more.

Is it possible you eat even when you don't need to?

Most of the time, we eat based on what our peers do. A lot of people eat visually, which means they try to eat everything on their plate or bowl, no matter what size it is. Some people never really feel hungry because their desire to eat keeps them full all the time. Hormones, sensations, or emotions can make you want to eat. This means enticing aromas, tastes, and sounds, or feelings such as stress, may tempt you even during your fasting period. True hunger, on the other hand, is a physical feeling, often accompanied by discomfort in the stomach and growling.

The hardest part of fasting is the beginning, when your cravings make you want to eat, and real hunger takes some time to get used to. Below are some tricks you can use to easily control the urge to eat when you don't need to.

- **Stay hydrated:** Dehydration can sometimes mimic hunger. Ensure you're adequately hydrated throughout your fasting period.
- **Mindful eating:** Eat mindfully when it's time to break your fast. Pay attention to your body's hunger cues and stop eating when you feel satiated.
- **Distraction:** Engage in activities or tasks that keep your mind occupied during fasting periods. Sometimes, hunger cues are more pronounced when you're focused on them.
- **Gradual adaptation:** If you're new to intermittent fasting, your body may take time to adapt to fasting periods. Start with shorter fasts and gradually extend them as your body becomes more accustomed.
- **Nutrient-dense meals:** When you do eat, choose nutrient-dense foods that provide lasting satiety and help stabilize blood sugar levels.

Keep in mind that hunger is natural during a fast and doesn't necessarily mean that something is wrong. It's a normal part of the fasting process, and as your body adjusts to this eating pattern, you may find that your hunger cues become easier to control over time.

CHALLENGES TO EXPECT

As with any route of personal growth and development, intermittent fasting is both exciting and fraught with its share of ups and downs. Let's look into some challenges you may face when starting this journey.

- **Hunger pangs:** Your fast days are going to be challenging, and hunger pangs may be one of those challenges. According to studies, people often experience hunger during the first few days of a fasting program (Wilhelmi de Toledo et al., 2019). These feelings represent your body's attempt to adapt to a new dietary routine. They are usually temporary and tend to diminish as your body adapts to the fasting routine. Staying hydrated and keeping busy can help you navigate these initial pangs.
- **Mood fluctuations:** You may be very aware that a hungry person is easily irritable. Studies have proven that having low blood sugar levels during fasting can sometimes lead to mood swings or irritability (Mongraw-Chaffin, et al., 2019). Your body is recalibrating its energy sources, and it's normal to feel a bit off-kilter at times. Another study shows that women reported stronger levels of accomplishment, pride, and self-control toward the end of the fasting period than they did at the

beginning, despite being more irritable (Watkins & Serpell, 2016).

- **Energy variations:** You may notice fluctuations in your energy levels, especially during the early stages of intermittent fasting. As your body becomes more efficient at using stored fat for energy, you'll likely experience more consistent energy throughout the day. Until then, pacing yourself and taking short breaks when needed can help you manage energy variations.

- **Social issues:** Social gatherings and mealtimes with family and friends may present challenges. Explaining your fasting schedule to loved ones and finding supportive environments can ease these social situations.

- **Physical adaptations:** Your body will undergo physical adaptations as it adjusts to intermittent fasting. These changes can include weight loss, improved metabolic markers, and reduced waist circumference. While these are positive outcomes, they may also necessitate adjustments to your wardrobe and self-image.

- **Long-term planning:** As you progress on your intermittent fasting journey, it's essential to consider long-term planning. How will you sustain this lifestyle change? What strategies will you employ to ensure intermittent fasting remains a practical and enjoyable part of your life? Of course, we are going to cover the best ideas on how to sustain it, but in the end, it will be up to you to determine your success and progress.

Intermittent fasting isn't a simple dietary choice; it's a transformative journey toward better health. The positive changes and benefits that manifest as you continue with intermittent fasting are the rewards of your commitment and resilience. You become the architect of your own wellness journey, shaping a future filled with vitality and triumph over the challenges of life.

KEY TAKEAWAYS

Intermittent fasting is an eating routine that involves cycling between periods of eating and fasting. It's not a diet per se, but rather a lifestyle adjustment that prioritizes the timing of your meals over the specific foods you eat. Intermittent fasting aligns with your body's natural circadian rhythms.

The science behind fasting:

- Intermittent fasting works by creating a calorie deficit during fasting periods, leading to weight loss.
- It enhances insulin sensitivity, promoting better blood sugar control.

Benefits of intermittent fasting:

- Intermittent fasting creates room for sustainable weight management and may reduce your risk of developing obesity-related diseases.
- It improves metabolic health, including insulin sensitivity and blood sugar regulation.
- Fasting affects metabolism, leading to improved energy utilization and fat breakdown.
- Intermittent fasting has a positive impact on your sleep, circadian rhythms, and hormonal balance.

The science of hunger:

- Hunger pangs during fasting are temporary and usually diminish as your body adapts to the routine.
- The practice of intermittent fasting promotes conscious eating and a healthier relationship with food.
- Sleep patterns may temporarily change when starting intermittent fasting, but they stabilize over time.
- Dehydration may affect your sleep quality during fasting, so proper hydration is crucial.

Challenges to expect:

- When starting intermittent fasting, you may struggle with issues such as hunger pangs and mood fluctuations.
- Increased alertness during fasting periods may interfere with your sleep, but your body will adjust as you continue your journey.
- Embracing flexibility and understanding your adjustment phase are key to success.

It's clear that the fundamentals of intermittent fasting offer a promising route to health and well-being, but keep in mind that your journey is also unique. It's fine if your method for intermittent fasting differs from what others are using.

In the next chapter, we'll go into the specifics of intermittent fasting techniques designed specifically to meet the special requirements of women in their 50s and beyond. These methods are not universal but are created to give you a specialized road map so you can maximize the benefits of intermittent fasting.

THREE LIFE-CHANGING STRATEGIES

Not all fasting methods work the same, especially for the discerning woman over 50. In a world full of fasting approaches, it's essential to discover strategies that suit your distinct requirements. As promised, we'll explore three life-changing intermittent fasting strategies specifically designed for women over 50. These strategies are both effective and considerate of the specific challenges and goals that you may have.

TIME-RESTRICTED EATING

Time-restricted eating (TRE) can be a highly effective approach, particularly if you are over 50. The approach is based on the idea that you should only eat during a specific window of time and fast for the rest of the time. For instance, you could have your meals within a 6 to 8-hour window, and then abstain from eating for the subsequent 16 to 18 hours of the day. This method depends on your body's circadian rhythms, which means that your meal times should match your body's natural clock.

The fasting part of TRE is when the magic happens. Remember, as we discussed in Chapter 2, that when your body doesn't get any food for a long time, it stops using glucose as fuel and starts burning fat in a process called ketosis. This shift helps with weight loss, keeping your hormones in balance, and improving your metabolism performance. Another beautiful thing about TRE is that it's flexible; it allows you to set your eating and fasting times so that they correspond with your daily schedule and personal preferences.

Let's explore the different types of TRE, covering the 16:8 and 18:6 approaches and what makes them special. I'll also give you useful tips on how to use TRE correctly so you can fully utilize its benefits to attain your health and fitness objectives.

The 16:8 Method

TRE has different fasting and eating windows, but we'll start with the 16:8 approach. It's one of the most popular methods and is easy to follow. We'll look into what this ratio means, how you can use it, and some real-life examples that will help paint a clear picture of what the strategy is all about.

The 16:8 method simply means that you eat for 8 hours and fast for about 16 hours. This fasting plan works for many women over 50 because it fits with their daily schedules and gives them a balanced way to do intermittent fasting.

The first step to implementing it is to pick your window. While choosing a window is totally a personal choice, I'll give an example of something I found effective. Consider picking your fasting hours from the evening until the next day. So, if you eat dinner at 7 p.m., you shouldn't eat anything until 11 a.m. the following day. You can only consume calorie-free beverages like water, herbal tea, and black coffee throughout the fasting period.

Next, you'll want to plan your meals right. You may eat two to three meals or snacks in your 8-hour eating window. To get the most out of your mealtime, try to focus on foods that are high in nutrients. Make sure you get the right amount of healthy fats, lean proteins, and carbohydrates.

Practical examples:

- If you're a morning person, you could start your fast after an early dinner, say at 6 p.m. You would then have your first meal around 10 a.m. the next day, which could be in time for your breakfast.
- If your evenings are more social or you prefer dinner with family, you could have your last meal

at 9 p.m. and fast until 1 p.m. the next day,
enjoying a satisfying lunch.

TRE is flexible, so you can adjust your eating window to suit your schedule. For example, you could have your first meal at 9 a.m. and finish your last meal by 5 p.m.

There are many women over 50 who like the 16:8 method because it gives them a balanced plan that works with their daily lives. It's not too strict and gives you room to be socially flexible while you still enjoy the benefits of fasting. Just be sure to pick a time range that works with your schedule and tastes.

The 18:6 Method

The 18:6 approach is another popular time-restricted eating pattern that's embraced by many. Let's explore what it consists of, how to effectively practice it, and some practical examples to guide you in implementing it.

With the 18:6 approach, you fast for 18 hours and eat within a 6-hour timeframe. This is ideal if you prefer longer fasting periods to short ones, but still want to eat within a day.

Many women who use this method choose their windows from the evening until the following morning or afternoon. For example, if you finish dinner by 8 p.m., your fasting period will extend until 2 p.m. the next day.

Next, you'll want to plan your meals, aiming for two to three well-balanced meals or snacks during your 6-hour eating window. To get the most out of your intermittent fasting approach, prioritize your nutrient-rich foods.

Practical examples:

- If you prefer an afternoon eating window, you may begin your fast after dinner at 6 p.m. and break it at 12 p.m. the next day with a nutritious lunch.
- Alternatively, if you find it more convenient to have your breakfast in the morning, you could have your last meal at 3 p.m. and break your fast at 9 a.m. with a balanced breakfast.

As long as you follow the 16:8 principle as explained, you can continue to adjust your fasting and eating windows until you find the best times for your daily routine.

Knowing when you naturally have the most energy also assists in figuring out the best times for fasting and eating. For example, if you usually feel more energetic in the morning, fasting during this time might feel easier for you and help you become more in sync with your body's natural patterns.

Tips for Successful Time-Restricted Eating

We have looked at the most common and suitable time-restricted eating patterns, but how can you put these patterns into practice effectively? Well, below I have some valuable tips that may help you succeed with TRE.

- **Take it slow:** If you're not familiar with intermittent fasting, it's best to gradually introduce yourself to TRE. You may begin by fasting for 12 hours and then gradually increase the fasting window as your body gets used to it.
- **Maintain sufficient hydration:** You need to make sure you look out for your health during your fasting period, as well as maintain sufficient hydration. Water, herbal tea, and black coffee are typically acceptable options to quench your thirst and they may also help ease your appetite.
- **Prioritize nutrition:** Make eating meals that are rich in nutrients a top priority. When it's time to eat, make sure to incorporate a variety of lean proteins, healthy fats, and some carbohydrates into your diet.
- **Listen to your body:** Make sure to pay attention to your body's hunger cues and energy levels. You might want to think about adjusting the length of your fast or looking into alternate fasting techniques if you're not feeling well or are overly hungry while you're fasting.

- **Be consistent:** Maintaining consistency is essential for success with TRE. In order to build a routine that works well with your everyday life, try to make your fasting and eating schedule fit perfectly with your life for consistency's sake.
- **Plan your meals in advance:** If you have a set eating window, it's a good idea to schedule your meals and snacks in advance. You may ensure that you're consuming a range of healthy and satiating foods this way. This can also help prevent making hasty and unhealthy decisions.
- **Exercise:** Be sure to include regular exercise in your daily routine. When planning your workouts, it's important to take your energy levels into account. While some women may find it more comfortable to exercise after their fast has ended, others may prefer to exercise while they are fasting.
- **Manage stress:** When it comes to fasting, managing stress is important. How you react to fasting may be impacted by ongoing stress. It's a good idea to integrate stress-reduction techniques into your daily routine to help improve your overall health. These methods include things like yoga, deep breathing exercises, and meditation.
- **Monitor your progress:** To document your TRE experience, you may want to consider writing in a diary. Please be aware of your mental and physical well-being, any changes in weight, and any other

pertinent observations. You can also record your progress using pictures or by measuring loss in inches, rather than relying on your scale only. This helps because muscle weighs more than fat, so you might think you are not making progress even when you are.

- **Patience:** Remember to have patience with yourself because results might not show up right away. TRE entails a change in lifestyle rather than a quick remedy. With time, you'll start noticing its advantages and enjoying the fruits of your hard work.

Disadvantages of Time-Restricted Eating

While TRE offers various intermittent fasting benefits, it's also important for you to know the potential disadvantages and when this fasting strategy requires caution.

- **Hunger and discomfort:** During the fasting window, particularly at first, you may feel very hungry and uncomfortable. This may result in irritability and trouble focusing.
- **Social difficulties:** It's a common human habit to have social events and mealtimes frequently outside of the fasting window. However, this makes it difficult to handle social gathering events, which may impact your social relationships and make maintaining TRE more

difficult. You may want to explain your new lifestyle to your family and friends in order to make this easier for you.

- **Risk of overeating:** If not well planned, there is a risk of overeating or making unwise food choices within the eating window. You may unknowingly consume a lot of calories when you're only trying to reward yourself.

Who Shouldn't Try Time-Restricted Eating

Before attempting TRE, if you live with any medical problems such as diabetes, eating disorders, anemia, or a history of hypoglycemia, you may want to consider talking to your healthcare professional before diving into it.

You may also need to factor in some medication considerations if you're on treatment. Some drugs require food consumption for optimal absorption, so it'd be wise to talk to your doctor about TRE to make sure it won't interfere with your regular dosage schedule or the mechanism of action of your medication.

ONE MEAL A DAY

You may have already done this once or twice, but unintentionally. I have noticed how some people may get busy and not think of food until their day is over. Sometimes, a person may only eat once a day, and when you use this approach as part of your intermittent fasting journey, it's called one meal a day (OMAD). This involves a very limited window to consume your meal, as you might expect. You fast for 23 hours each day, then have a single meal that contains all the calories you need for the day. It's important to nourish yourself during the fasting period with noncaloric beverages such as water, herbal tea, or black coffee.

It's also crucial to take into account that your one meal should be nutrient-dense and balanced to ensure that you meet your daily nutritional needs. During your 23 hours of fasting, there are some metabolic shifts that occur. These processes play a fundamental role in helping your body adapt to the extended fasting window of OMAD.

Remember, when you first start fasting, your body relies on glycogen stores in the liver and muscles for energy. Glycogen is the form of glucose that is stored in the body, and these glycogen reserves deplete within 12 to 18 hours of fasting. Once glycogen stores are used up, your body shifts its primary energy source from glucose to stored fat. This transition is a key aspect of longer fasts and the OMAD approach. After about 18 hours of fasting, your body enters ketosis, the process in which the liver produces molecules called ketones from fat breakdown. Ketones become the primary source of energy, particularly for the brain. This metabolic shift helps preserve muscle mass while burning fat for fuel.

Benefits of One Meal a Day

- **Simplicity:** With OMAD, fasting becomes effortless. You can wave goodbye to complicated meal planning and the hassle of juggling multiple eating windows throughout the day.
- **Deeper ketosis state:** When you extend your fasting time to OMAD, it can potentially lead to experiencing deeper states of ketosis. This means that your body becomes more proficient at using stored fat as a source of energy, leading to enhanced fat burning and achieving a more toned physique.
- **Muscle mass preservation:** When it comes to preserving muscle mass, prolonged fasting in OMAD has an advantage over some other fasting methods. Our bodies have a natural inclination to prioritize the breakdown of fat rather than muscle tissue.
- **Appetite suppression:** One of the great things about prolonged fasting is that it naturally helps to suppress your appetite. Remember the hormone ghrelin, which is responsible for triggering hunger? It tends to decrease during prolonged fasting periods like OMAD. This makes it more manageable to stick to for longer fasting periods.
- **Increased autophagy:** When you fast for longer periods, it can actually boost autophagy, which, as

you'll recall, has the potential to promote cellular health and rejuvenation.

- **Improved insulin sensitivity:** We covered this as one of the advantages of IF, and engaging OMAD practice may further reduce your chances of developing insulin resistance and type 2 diabetes.

Disadvantages of the One Meal a Day Approach

- **Extreme nature:** OMAD is an intense fasting regimen that may not be suitable for everyone. The extended fasting period can lead to hunger, low energy levels, and potential difficulties in adhering to the plan in the beginning. This may have an impact on daily activities and general health.
- **Nutrient deficiency:** Consuming all your daily calories in one meal may make it challenging to ensure adequate nutrient intake. Being a woman over 50 will require you to have essential vitamins and minerals for bone health, hormonal balance, and overall well-being. Careful meal planning is essential to prevent nutrient deficiencies.
- **Digestive challenges:** A large, calorie-dense meal in a short time frame may place stress on the digestive system, potentially leading to discomfort, bloating, or digestive issues, which can be more pronounced with age.

- **Potential for overeating:** While OMAD can lead to calorie restriction, it also carries the risk of overeating during the single meal, which may negate potential weight loss benefits.
- **Social and lifestyle impact:** OMAD can affect social interactions and mealtime traditions, which may be important if you are a woman who values shared meals with family and friends. It can also limit flexibility in daily routines.
- **Effect on medications:** If you are taking medications, you may need to adjust your eating time to align with the medication timing as some medications require food intake for proper absorption.
- **Hydration concerns:** Extended fasting periods can lead to dehydration if fluid intake is not adequately managed. Hydration is a must, especially during fasting.
- **Potential stress:** Some women feel stressed, particularly if they feel pressured to meet their daily nutritional needs within a single meal.
- **Individual variability:** OMAD is not suitable for everyone, and some people do not respond to it in a positive way.

Success Tips for the One Meal-a-Day Approach

- **Meal planning and prioritizing nutrient density:** Plan your meal thoughtfully to ensure it's balanced and provides essential nutrients. Focus on lean proteins, healthy fats, whole grains, plenty of fruits and vegetables, and dairy or dairy alternatives to meet your nutritional needs. You might want to think about seeking the individualized meal-planning advice of a licensed dietitian.
- **Hydration:** Stay adequately hydrated throughout the fasting period until you have your meal. Drinking water, herbal tea, or black coffee can help curb hunger and maintain hydration levels.
- **Gradual transition:** If you're new to OMAD, you may want to consider a gradual transition. A practical approach is beginning with shorter fasting windows, like 16:8 or 18:6, and then slowly extending the fasting duration as your body adjusts.
- **Listening to your body:** Watch out for signs that you're hungry and listen to your body. It's okay to change your fasting window or meal times if you feel too tired or hungry.
- **Monitoring medications:** If you take medications, work with your healthcare provider to adjust medication timing as needed to accommodate OMAD.

- **Social flexibility:** Even though OMAD might make social meals harder, try to find a way to still eat with family and friends every once in a while.
- **Mindful eating:** After a long 23 hours of fasting, it may be hard to mindfully eat, but you should strive to practice mindful eating during your OMAD meal. You can achieve this by chewing each bite thoroughly and concentrating on the meal's sensory experience. This helps prevent overeating.
- **Staying consistent:** Consistency is key to success with everything you do. Try to maintain a consistent eating window and mealtime to regulate your body's internal clock.
- **Regular physical activity:** Adding regular physical exercise to your schedule can help your health and well-being as a whole. Working out can add to the perks of OMAD.
- **Health monitoring:** Regularly monitor your health, including your blood sugar levels. Keep track of any changes and discuss them with your healthcare provider.
- **Seeking professional guidance:** Talk to your doctor and a qualified dietitian to make sure that OMAD is right for your health and to get advice from professionals.

It's essential for you to approach OMAD with careful consideration of your unique health needs and goals.

Consulting with a healthcare provider and a registered dietitian is advisable to ensure that OMAD aligns with your health profiles and is carried out safely and effectively. It may also be beneficial to explore alternative fasting methods, such as time-restricted eating or modified fasting regimens, to find an approach that best suits your individual preferences and needs.

5:2 DIET

The 5:2 diet, commonly referred to as the fast diet, is based on eating normally five days a week while significantly reducing calorie intake on the other two days that aren't consecutive. Typically, during these two fasting days, which are often referred to as restrictive days, you would aim for an intake of about 500 to 600 calories per day on average.

One thing that makes the 5:2 diet unique and easy to follow is that it doesn't require fasting every day or for a long period of time. The 5:2 diet differs from TRE in that it's primarily centered on calorie restriction while TRE focuses on narrowing the window of time during which you eat each day.

Although this approach doesn't always provide the same fasting benefits as TRE, such as autophagy or deep ketosis, it has its own health advantages. If you are a woman with a busy schedule, this method gives you the freedom to pick which days to set aside as restriction days based on your own plan and preferences. Because it's flexible, it's easy to work into different routines.

Success Tips for the 5:2 Diet

The 5:2 diet strikes a balance between achieving fasting benefits and maintaining a practical and sustainable approach when you are over 50. Eating on fasting days during the 5:2 method requires careful planning to ensure you meet your nutritional needs while adhering to the calorie restriction. Here are some tips on how to eat when using this approach:

- **Choose nutrient-dense foods:** Choose foods that give you the vitamins and minerals you need without adding a lot of calories. Eat lots of whole grains, veggies, and lean proteins. These foods can make you feel full and give you the nutrients you need.
- **Stay hydrated:** Drink a lot of water throughout the day to stay hydrated. Herbal tea or black coffee (without sugar or cream) can also be consumed to curb hunger.
- **Divide calories wisely:** On fasting days, you can only eat a certain number of calories, so it's important to plan how you eat them. You have the flexibility to have a small breakfast, lunch, and dinner on those days, or you can choose to incorporate snacks during the day.

- **Include protein:** Protein helps maintain muscle mass and keeps you feeling full. You may opt for lean protein such as chicken or legumes.
- **Add some fiber:** High-fiber foods like vegetables, whole grains, and legumes may help control hunger and stabilize blood sugar levels.
- **Limit sugars and refined carbs:** Avoid sugary snacks and refined carbohydrates, as they can lead to rapid blood sugar spikes and crashes, which may exacerbate hunger.
- **Watch portion sizes:** Be mindful of portion sizes to ensure you stay within your calorie limit. You may think of using measuring cups or a food scale if necessary.
- **Avoid high-calorie condiments:** You may not be aware, but some sauces, dressings, and condiments can add extra calories faster than you think. You may want to use low-calorie or homemade options.
- **Listen to your body:** Pay attention to signs that you're hungry. If you're feeling really hungry, you can change when you eat or snack.
- **Plan ahead:** Plan your meals for fasting days in advance. Making better decisions and staying on track will be easier if you have a clear plan.
- **Consider intermittent fasting apps:** There are several mobile apps available that can help you track your fasting days, count calories, and plan meals effectively.

Real-Life Success Story With 5:2

Here is an encouraging story from another woman like you and me who can testify to the effectiveness of intermittent fasting:

A few years back, I successfully shed 125 lbs., largely thanks to the 16:8 intermittent fasting method. However, when the pandemic hit and my life underwent significant changes, I found it challenging to stick to the 16:8 routine and regained some of the weight.

In search of a more compatible approach, I gave 5:2 fasting a try, and it's been nothing short of amazing. This method aligns better with my eating habits and mindset. On five days of the week, I consume maintenance calories, totaling 2400 calories. It feels like I'm almost having a "cheat day" each of those days, and this calorie allowance also sustains me during late-night hockey games when I need the energy. Restricting myself to 1800–2000 calories made it tough to maintain my energy levels.

On the other two days, I limit my intake to 600 calories, essentially having one meal a day. Surprisingly, these days have been quite manageable because I view them as a prelude to a 2,400-calorie day right after. Moreover, these 600-calorie days help me regain my focus, eliminating any guilt I might feel after occasional overindulgence.

In just three weeks, I've shed over 10 lbs., with a significant portion of that being an initial rapid loss. The best part is that it has felt nearly effortless. It's essential to remember that fasting methods vary in effectiveness from person to person, so 5:2 might not be the ideal fit for everyone. All you have to do is to adapt your intermittent fasting routine to suit your current lifestyle while leaving room to try new strategies that'll make your eating approach more fun.

OTHER INTERMITTENT FASTING APPROACHES

Let's look into other intermittent fasting options that we haven't covered yet:

- **The warrior diet:** With the warrior diet, you adhere to a 20:4 fasting pattern. This involves fasting for 20 hours and having a four-hour eating window. You consume tiny amounts of fresh fruits and vegetables throughout the fasting hours and keep your big meal for the 4-hour window. This strategy is based on the eating habits of ancient warriors and emphasizes eating at night. It may be appealing if you prefer larger, more filling evening meals.

- **Weekly 24-hour fast:** This method entails fasting for a complete 24 hours once a week. For instance, you could begin your fast after dinner one day and end it with dinner the next. Although this strategy helps reset your eating patterns and calorie intake for the week, it's less frequent than other intermittent fasting methods.
- **Alternate day fasting:** This method alternates between fasting days and regular eating days. On fasting days, you consume extremely little or no calories, whereas on eating days, you eat normally. On fasting days, some varieties allow for a limited number of calories. This method can be difficult, but it can result in considerable calorie deficits and weight loss.
- **12 hours fast each day:** The 12:12 approach, as this practice is commonly known, calls for a 12-hour fast followed by 12 hours of eating. It's one of the most basic types of intermittent fasting, and you may incorporate it into your everyday routine simply by modifying your meal times. For example, you may eat breakfast at 7 a.m. and dinner at 7 p.m., resulting in a 12-hour fasting period overnight.

Finding a sustainable method that fits your lifestyle and supports your health goals is what determines your success with intermittent fasting.

KEY TAKEAWAYS

Time-restricted eating: the 16:8 and 18:6 methods

- Time-restricted eating involves limiting your eating to specific time windows during the day.
- The 16:8 method allows for an 8-hour eating window and a 16-hour fasting period.
- The 18:6 diet provides a 6-hour window for eating and an 18-hour window for fasting.
- These methods provide simplicity and flexibility, making them suitable for beginners.
- These strategies can assist in regulating your calorie intake and fostering weight loss.

The one meal-a-day approach:

- OMAD entails consuming all daily calories in one meal, typically within a 1-hour eating window.
- This approach is considered an intense form of intermittent fasting and may result in substantial calorie deficits.
- Longer fasting periods leading up to the OMAD meal may enhance metabolic effects.
- Potential benefits include deeper ketosis and increased autophagy.
- Nutrient density is crucial when following OMAD to meet nutritional needs.

5:2 diet

- The 5:2 diet consists of rotating between 5 non-fasting days and 2 fasting days each week.
- During fasting days, you restrict your calorie intake to approximately 500–600 calories.
- This method is less stringent than daily fasting and can be easier to maintain.
- It can fit seamlessly into a weekly routine and offers flexibility.
- On non-fasting days, it's essential not to exceed the recommended daily calorie intake.

Other intermittent fasting approaches

- The warrior diet follows a 20:4 fasting schedule with a 4-hour eating window in the evening.
- Weekly 24-hour fasting involves fasting for a full 24 hours once a week.
- Alternate day fasting involves switching between fasting days and normal eating days.
- Fasting for 12 hours a day (12:12) is a simple method involving a 12-hour fasting period and a 12-hour eating window.

The choice of an intermittent fasting method should align with your individual preferences, lifestyle, and health goals.

These intermittent fasting methods offer various options for achieving calorie reduction, promoting weight loss, and supporting overall health. Your particular needs and personal preferences should be taken into consideration while deciding which approach to use. As with any dietary changes, it's advisable to seek guidance from a healthcare provider or registered dietitian, especially if you have underlying medical conditions or specific dietary requirements.

As we wrap up this chapter, I would like you to remember that while the choice of fasting method is important, the nutritional quality of your meals within those eating windows is paramount. The benefits of intermittent fasting are tightly intertwined with the nutrients you consume. In the next chapter, we'll focus on nutrition during intermittent fasting, and I'll share some secrets to optimizing your fasting experience. You will discover the science behind nutrient needs during fasting and how to use this knowledge to unlock the full potential of inter-mittent fasting for your health and well-being.

4

NUTRITION: FUELING THE FASTING BODY

Ever wondered why two people can fast in the same way, following the same regimen, and yet achieve vastly different results? The answer lies in the tangled relationship between nutrition and intermittent fasting. In this chapter, we'll explore the important role that nutrition plays in your body. You'll gain a deep understanding of how to nourish your body adequately during fasting periods, ensuring that your efforts yield the best possible outcomes.

MACRONUTRIENTS AND MICRONUTRIENTS

When you think about eating healthily, think of nutrition. Nutrition encompasses everything you eat and drink to sustain your body. There are typically two major divisions: macronutrients and micronutrients. Let's take a closer look at these categories and the role they play when fasting.

Macronutrients

Macronutrients help provide your body with energy in order for you to sustain activities your body undertakes. They consist of three primary components:

- **Carbohydrates:** Remember, your body breaks carbohydrates down into glucose to fuel up your cells. These serve as the body's main energy sources. You can obtain them from healthy foods that include vegetables or whole grains, as well as unhealthy foods like cookies and muffins. This is why they have an unfavorable perception in some diets. We can further divide this class of macronutrients into simple and complex carbohydrates. The two differ because of the chemical makeup each contains, which changes how quickly the body absorbs the sugar. Processed and refined sugars are used to create simple carbohydrates, lacking essential vitamins, minerals, and proteins. As a result, the simple form tends to release sugar more quickly, meaning the body will also consume it fast. Complex carbohydrates, also called good carbs, break down more slowly and are full of different nutrients. Each gram of carbohydrates contains about 4 calories, which is important when you want to keep track of how many calories you consume in a meal.

- **Proteins:** Proteins are known as the building blocks of the body and are made from amino acids. They have the ability to build and fix your body tissues. Proteins are also found in hair, skin, and muscle fibers and contribute to the production of enzymes and hormones. Proteins do not provide direct energy but help build other parts of your body. How healthy a protein is depends on how many essential amino acids it has, which differs according to the source of the protein. All essential amino acids are present in meat or fish. Consuming adequate protein helps keep hunger hormones in check, which explains why meals that are high in protein tend to make you less hungry. About 4 calories are contained in every gram of protein. When fasting, proteins help you maintain your muscle mass and ensure your body always has enough amino acids for its important functions.

- **Fats:** Also known as lipids, fats supply energy in small amounts per unit mass. Fats provide approximately 9 calories per gram. They also promote cell proliferation and are crucial for the uptake of fat-soluble nutrients. They include saturated, unsaturated, and trans fat. It's important to know the difference between saturated and unsaturated fats. Unsaturated fats help maintain cell membrane structure, control metabolism, and help cells grow and repair themselves. They also facilitate the absorption of fat-soluble vitamins A, D, E, and K. Although your body doesn't need saturated fats, they help provide you with cholesterol, which is important when producing hormones. Your body makes cholesterol itself, but can also benefit a small amount from food. Cholesterol helps build cell membranes, speed up your metabolism, and make bile acids, which help break down fats and obtain nutrients. On the flip side, consuming a meal that's rich in cholesterol raises your chances of developing heart disease.

It's very important to balance these macronutrients while fasting. This may help you control your hormones, keep your energy up, and stay healthy while you're fasting.

The precise amounts of macronutrients vary for each person and rely on your age-related fundamental needs, your level of physical activity, and your weight loss objectives. The following are the suggested macronutrient estimates provided by the Dietary Guidelines for Americans (USDA, 2015).

- 45 to 65% of calories from carbohydrates
- 20 to 35% of calories from fat

- 10 to 35% of calories from proteins

Studies show that a woman should aim to consume no more than 1,500 calories per day in order to shed one pound per week, and no more than 2,000 calories per day on average in order to maintain her weight (Osilla et al., 2020).

A macro-counting diet starts with calculating daily calorie needs. This will be entirely based on your goals, on which you will also decide what certain percentage of calories to eat from each food group. For example, if your aim is to build muscles, you may take more protein to help with that but if your aim is to regulate your blood sugar levels, then you may eat fewer carbohydrates.

Micronutrients

Your body requires micronutrients in specified amounts in order to function properly. Even though you may only need small amounts of them compared to macronutrients like proteins and carbohydrates, micronutrients are very important for staying healthy and avoiding many diseases and deficiencies. Micronutrients are mostly broken down into two groups: vitamins and minerals.

Vitamins

Vitamins are organic substances that the body needs to complete many complex biological processes. Vitamins come in various forms, and they can be categorized into two main groups: water-soluble vitamins, such as vitamin C and the B-complex vitamins, and fat-soluble vitamins, which include vitamins A, D, E, and K. Each vitamin has its own function.

- **Vitamin A:** Getting enough vitamin A is important for keeping your eyes healthy, and your immune system strong. Vitamin A also helps cells divide and split into new cells, contributing to growth and development. Vitamin A is found in carrots, sweet potatoes, spinach, and liver.
- **Vitamin B:** The B vitamins, examples include thiamine, riboflavin, niacin, and folate, help the body make energy, maintain nerve health, and aid in breaking down macronutrients. Red blood cell formation and DNA replication depend on B vitamins. B vitamins are abundant in whole grains, legumes, nuts, and leafy green vegetables.
- **Vitamin C:** Also referred to as ascorbic acid, vitamin C is a potent antioxidant that shields cells from harm inflicted by free radicals. Free radicals are atoms that aren't stable and are capable of damaging cells, which may result in you being ill or speeding up the aging process. Your body

requires vitamin C to make *collagen*, a protein that helps cuts heal and keeps skin, bones, and blood vessels healthy. Vitamin C also helps in strengthening your immune system. This vitamin is abundant in citrus fruits, strawberries, bell peppers, and broccoli.

- **Vitamin D:** Vitamin D is excellent for maintaining the health and strength of your skin, hair, and nails, as it supports cell growth and differentiation in these tissues. Vitamin D also helps the body make keratin, a protein that is important for the structure of our skin, hair, and nails. Fatty fish, fortified dairy products, and sun exposure are good sources of vitamin D.

- **Vitamin E:** This acts as an antioxidant, safeguarding your cells against damage caused by free radicals and contributing to the repair of skin cells, which can help maintain a youthful appearance. You can find vitamin E in nuts, seeds, vegetable oils, and leafy green vegetables.

- **Vitamin K:** Vitamin K plays a vital role in blood clotting and bone health. It activates proteins that aid in blood clotting to prevent excessive bleeding, and it's essential for proper calcium absorption, which is crucial for maintaining strong bones. Leafy green vegetables, broccoli, and brussels sprouts are good sources of vitamin K.

Minerals

Minerals are inorganic nutrients important for maintaining healthy bones, fluid equilibrium, neuron function, and other processes. Let's discuss some common minerals and their function:

- **Calcium:** Calcium is essential for maintaining strong bones and teeth because it helps build and maintain the structure of these tissues. Additionally, it plays a critical role in muscle function by assisting in muscle contractions. Calcium is involved in nerve transmission, allowing for the communication between nerve cells. It is also important for hormone secretion, which helps regulate various bodily functions. Furthermore, it plays a role in blood clotting, preventing excessive bleeding, and helps regulate blood pressure, supporting cardiovascular health. Calcium is found in dairy products and if you follow a plant-based diet, sources of calcium include dairy alternatives such as fortified plant-based milk, tofu, and leafy greens like kale and broccoli.
- **Zinc:** Zinc is important for a healthy immune system, as it helps in the production of immune cells and supports their proper functioning. Additionally, it aids in cell division, DNA synthesis, and the healing of wounds. Zinc is

involved in taste and smell perception, as well as in maintaining healthy skin and hair. A deficiency in zinc may weaken your immune system, making you more susceptible to infections and illnesses. Additionally, it may result in slower wound recovery and a loss of taste and smell. A lack of zinc affects skin and hair health, resulting in conditions such as dry skin and hair loss. Some sources of this mineral include oysters, beef, and poultry. If you prefer plant-based diets, you can also obtain zinc from legumes, nuts, and seeds, as well as fortified cereals.

- **Magnesium:** This is essential for numerous bodily functions, including energy production, muscle contraction, and nerve function. Magnesium is also essential for maintaining a healthy heart rhythm and promoting bone health. Furthermore, it aids in controlling blood sugar levels and participates in the synthesis of DNA and proteins. Consuming foods that contain the mineral in the right amounts promotes relaxation and improves sleep quality. A deficiency in magnesium can lead to muscle weakness, cramps, and impaired nerve function. It can also increase the risk of heart rhythm abnormalities and negatively impact bone health. Magnesium is found in leafy green vegetables, nuts, seeds, and whole grains.

- **Iron:** Iron is a vital mineral that is essential for creating hemoglobin, a protein within red blood

cells that transports oxygen throughout your
body. It also plays a crucial part in energy
generation and metabolism. Moreover, iron is
essential for supporting a robust immune system
and cognitive abilities. If you lack iron, you may
experience fatigue, weakness, and reduced
immunity. To meet your body's iron
requirements, focus on consuming iron-rich
foods such as red meat, spinach, lentils, and
fortified cereals.

Making sure you get enough of these nutrients is important for your health during intermittent fasting. If you
don't do it right, fasting can leave you lacking in nutrients,
and this may lead to some of the health concerns we have
covered.

The Importance of Micronutrients for Women Over 50

We have already discussed how our hormones become
unbalanced during menopause. Fortunately, micronutrients, such as magnesium, play a role in hormonal regulation. Magnesium helps alleviate symptoms related to
hormonal fluctuations, such as mood swings and sleep
disturbances.

There are many other reasons it's important for you to
consume enough micronutrients, and here are some of
them:

- **Bone health:** Women over 50 are at a higher risk of bone density loss, leading to conditions such as osteoporosis, which can make your bones fragile and easy to break. Micronutrients such as calcium and vitamin D are crucial for maintaining bone strength and reducing the risk of fractures. Maintaining sufficient intake of these nutrients is crucial for supporting the health of your bones.
- **Immune function:** As you age, your immune system becomes less efficient in fighting off diseases and repairing cells. Adequate micronutrient intake, including vitamin C and zinc, is vital to support immune function. These micronutrients can help your body defend itself against infections and illnesses, which is definitely a benefit for your aging immune system.
- **Vision and skin health:** It's well known that aging brings changes in vision and skin health. Maintaining healthy skin and eyesight requires vitamin A. Vitamin E is another micronutrient that may help preserve your skin health.

HOW TO BREAK A FAST: FOODS TO OPT FOR AND FOODS TO AVOID

Now that you understand what nutrition is and which foods provide the essential nutrients during your eating window, we'll explore how to break a fast. You may wonder if there are rules to breaking a fast or if one can eat whatever they want, so here is a list of some foods to opt for, and which ones to avoid when breaking a fast.

Foods for Breaking a Fast

It's important to choose foods that are gentle on your digestive system. When breaking a fast, you should opt for foods that contain essential nutrients but won't overwhelm the stomach. Below is a list of some foods that would be of help when breaking a fast:

- **Bone broth:** This is perfect to break a fast because it's gentle on the stomach and can be taken during that transitional period after fasting. It also has lots of nutrients, such as collagen and amino acids that are beneficial to gut health.
- **Lean protein:** Your body uses amino acids as a repair and building tool, especially if you have exercised while fasting. Lean protein provides these amino acids to your diet to aid muscle recovery. You can find lean protein from sources like chicken, turkey, fish, or legumes if you are on a plant-based diet.
- **Fibrous vegetables:** Non-starchy vegetables like broccoli, spinach, and cauliflower, rich with fiber, provide essential vitamins and minerals. These assist in digestion and do not cause sudden blood spikes.

- **Healthy fats:** Such foods as avocados, nuts, and olive oil, which are rich in healthy fats, prove useful in ensuring satiety and improved general health. They provide a steady source of energy and support fat metabolism, which aligns with the goals of some fasting methods.
- **Complex carbohydrates:** Also known as good carbs, these are a good option because they release energy slowly and maintain stable blood sugar levels. Some sources include whole grains, quinoa, and sweet potatoes.
- **Fermented foods:** These may include yogurt, kefir, or sauerkraut, which are all rich in probiotics and thus support good gut health.

Foods to Avoid When Breaking a Fast

Some foods can be harsh on an empty stomach or cause rapid spikes in blood sugar. Here is a list of some foods to avoid:

- **Highly processed foods:** You should try by all means necessary to avoid highly processed food such as sugary cereal, fast foods, or other prepackaged food. Such food items are rich in refined sugars, unhealthy fats, and chemical contents that lead to blood sugar rise and digestive problems.

- **Greasy, fried foods:** Greasy and deep-fried foods like fried chicken and fries, cheeseburgers, or onion rings, are difficult to break down and may lead to indigestion, especially when your digestive system is just waking up from a fast.
- **Spicy foods:** Sometimes, it's unavoidable not to add spice to your food. However, extremely spicy meals may irritate your stomach and cause discomfort or heartburn, which are undesirable when fasting.
- **Excessive alcohol:** When taken on an empty stomach, alcohol can be harsh on an empty stomach and may lead to rapid intoxication. Try staying away from alcohol when breaking a fast and if you are unsure how your body will respond.
- **Simple carbohydrates:** You should also avoid consuming processed or refined carbohydrate-rich foods such as white breads, sugary cereals, chocolates, sodas, or sweets. These cause an abrupt increase in blood sugar levels and then a crash that makes you feel weak and famished.

Avoiding these foods when breaking a fast helps prevent digestive discomfort, energy fluctuations, and other issues that might negate the benefits of your fasting period. Nutrient-dense, balanced meals are the only way to go!

SUPPLEMENTS: ARE THEY NECESSARY?

I cannot emphasize enough that whole foods are ideal in terms of nutrition because they offer a wide variety of nutrients in their pure forms, often along with fiber and other advantageous elements. However, there are some circumstances in which supplements can benefit your fasting experience and general health. Here are several circumstances where you might need to think about taking supplements:

- **Nutrient gaps:** Despite your best efforts to maintain a balanced diet, it's possible to have nutrient gaps, especially when you're following a specific eating pattern like intermittent fasting. In such cases, supplements help bridge those gaps and ensure you're meeting your nutritional needs.
- **Specific health goals:** If you have certain targets for your health, such as supporting bone health, improving skin quality, anemia, or enhancing cognitive function, targeted supplements provide additional support. For example, calcium and vitamin D supplements are beneficial for bone health.

Below is a list of some supplements that are of interest during perimenopause and menopause:

- Vitamin A
- B vitamins
- Vitamin D
- Calcium
- Magnesium

We already covered the examples above and discussed their functions under micronutrients. Other supplements you may also need include these:

- **Omega-3:** Omega-3 helps lower inflammation and enhance heart function. Seafood-free diets might benefit from omega-3 tablets.
- **Probiotics:** Probiotics may help digestion and nutrition. Adding these supplements may help balance your gut bacteria.
- **Collagen:** Skin and joint collagen supplements are popular sources of additional collagen. They may reduce joint discomfort and age-related skin changes.

It's important to note that supplement needs may vary from woman to woman. Feel free to consult with a health-care provider or a registered dietitian to determine which supplements, if any, are suitable for your specific health goals and lifestyle needs.

How to Choose High-Quality Supplements

Picking quality supplements for the first time can be tricky because you may not know where to start. While I won't suggest specific brands for you, I'll share some hints to make sure your choice is of a high quality:

- **Look for third-party testing:** Choose supplements that have undergone third-party testing for quality and purity. Organizations like NSF International, USP, and ConsumerLab provide rigorous testing and certification.
- **Check for bioavailability:** Opt for supplements in forms that are highly bioavailable and easily absorbed by the body. For example, choose calcium citrate over calcium carbonate for better absorption.
- **Avoid artificial additives:** Check the ingredient list for artificial colors, preservatives, and fillers. High-quality supplements should contain minimal additional ingredients.
- **Consider allergens:** If you have allergies or sensitivities, check for common allergens in the supplement, such as gluten, soy, or dairy. Choose allergen-free options if needed.

Consult your healthcare professional before using any new supplement, particularly if you have certain health issues or are taking medication. In addition to making sure there are no possible interactions, they also offer individualized advice.

Timing of Supplements in Relation to Fasting

The following are tips on what time you should take your supplements while following intermittent fasting:

- **With meals:** In most cases, it's advisable to take supplements with meals or during your eating window. This can enhance the absorption of fat-soluble vitamins and minimize the risk of digestive discomfort (Fletcher, 2019). For example, take your vitamin D or omega-3 supplement with breakfast or lunch.
- **Fasting window:** Some supplements can be taken during your fasting window without breaking the fast. These typically include noncaloric supplements like certain vitamins and minerals. For instance, you can safely take a magnesium supplement during your fasting period.
- **Electrolytes:** During fasting, it's crucial to pay attention to your electrolyte balance. Electrolytes like sodium, potassium, and magnesium play a significant role in maintaining proper hydration and overall health. If you're concerned about electrolyte imbalances during fasting, consider using electrolyte supplements as needed. These supplements help ensure that you maintain the

right levels of these essential minerals, especially when fasting for extended periods.

- **Avoid sugar-containing supplements:** Steer clear of supplements that contain added sugars, as these can spike blood sugar levels and break your fast. Read labels carefully to ensure the supplements are sugar-free.
- **Customize to your schedule:** Adjust your supplement schedule to align with your fasting routine. For instance, if you practice a 16:8 fast and eat between 12 p.m. and 8 p.m., take supplements with your meals or during this window to maximize absorption.

HYDRATION: THE OFTEN-OVERLOOKED COMPONENT

Fasting can occasionally cause the perception of hunger when your body actually craves fluids. The role of water during intermittent fasting is sometimes ignored, although it is critical to a healthy fasting experience. Here's why staying hydrated is so important:

- **Hunger and thirst:** Feelings of hunger can come from not drinking enough water, which can make you break your fast early. Consider having a glass of water before your meal to help control your appetite. A simple sip can sometimes make you feel better when you're hungry.

- **Improved digestion:** Water helps your body process food, and if you go without food for a while, your bowel movements may change temporarily. Staying hydrated can help keep your digestive system healthy and running smoothly.
- **Energy levels:** People who are dehydrated may feel tired and sluggish, which can be mistaken for fatigue caused by fasting. Staying hydrated will help you keep up your energy levels while you're fasting.
- **Brain function:** Staying hydrated is important for brain health. Dehydration makes it hard to focus and causes mood swings, which could make fasting less enjoyable.
- **Controlled hunger:** During your fasting time, drinking water can help you control your hunger. It makes your stomach bigger, which tells your brain that you're full, which can be especially helpful if you're fasting for a long time.
- **Electrolyte balance:** Water helps with balancing electrolytes in the body by serving as a medium for their transportation. Electrolytes, such as sodium, potassium, and chloride, are dissolved in water and carried throughout the body to maintain proper fluid balance and facilitate nerve and muscle function. Staying hydrated with water supports the optimal functioning of electrolytes and prevents imbalances that may lead to dehydration or other health issues.

- **Enhanced cellular detoxification:** Adequate hydration aids in the removal of waste products and toxins from your cells.
- **Liver function:** Maintaining good hydration supports the proper function of your liver, which is essential for detoxifying your body by processing and eliminating toxins. Sufficient hydration helps the liver function optimally.
- **Kidney function:** Your kidneys serve the vital role of filtering waste and removing excess substances from your bloodstream. Proper hydration ensures the kidneys can efficiently remove metabolic waste products and maintain electrolyte balance.
- **Lymphatic system support:** Staying well-hydrated supports your lymphatic system, a crucial component of your body's immune and detoxification processes. A well-hydrated body ensures that lymph fluid can flow effectively, carrying away waste and pathogens.
- **Skin health:** Sufficient hydration is a contributing factor to maintaining healthy, glowing skin. The skin is an important part of the body's detoxification system. Proper hydration can support the skin's role in eliminating toxins through sweat.
- **Reduced risk of constipation:** Staying hydrated helps prevent constipation, which can be common during fasting. Adequate water intake keeps the

digestive system functioning smoothly, aiding in the elimination of waste.

Tips on Optimal Hydration and Electrolyte Balance During Fasting

Let's look at what you can drink while you are fasting below.

- **Water:** You probably guessed it, but water is the first on the list. It's easily accessible and the most important liquid for your body. You should aim to consume at least 8 to 10 glasses of water each day. You can easily adjust this based on personal needs if you need more than the minimum.
- **Herbal teas:** Teas such as chamomile, mint, or ginger from herbs can be a great way to add variety to your fluid intake.
- **Electrolytes:** If you're fasting for an extended period, consider adding a pinch of sea salt to your water or mineral water with added electrolytes. Low-sodium broths or bouillon cubes are another excellent choice because they provide a quick and easy source of sodium and other minerals. These essential minerals help prevent dehydration and maintain the balance your body needs for various functions.
- **Lemon water:** Adding a slice of lemon to your water can make the taste more enjoyable. Plus,

lemon water can also provide a slight electrolyte boost.

- **Coconut water:** Coconut water serves as a natural provider of electrolytes and a hydrating option during non-fasting days or within meal windows. It's especially useful for replacing minerals after physical activity or for extended fasts.
- **Limit caffeine:** While some caffeine can be part of your fasting practice, too much caffeine might dehydrate you. Consume coffee and tea in moderation and alternate with water.

Remember that everyone's water demands vary, so tailor these techniques to your own requirements and fasting pattern. Staying hydrated is essential for effective intermittent fasting, as it ensures you feel your best and reap the maximum advantages of your fasting schedule.

KEY TAKEAWAYS

Macronutrients and micronutrients:

- Macronutrients include carbohydrates, proteins, and fats, while micronutrients encompass vitamins and minerals.
- Each macronutrient has a specific role during fasting, impacting energy, hormone regulation, and overall health.

- Micronutrients are essential for bone health, immunity, and hormonal balance, making them crucial for women over 50.

How to break a fast:

- The post-fast meal can either maximize the benefits of fasting or negate them.
- Beneficial foods for breaking a fast include lean proteins, leafy greens, berries, nuts, and whole grains.
- Foods to avoid post-fast are those that can be harsh on an empty stomach or cause rapid blood sugar spikes.

Supplements:

- Supplements can complement fasting, but whole foods are excellent for your body.
- Choose high-quality supplements and time their consumption appropriately.

Hydration:

- Hydration is especially important during fasting because it's common to mistake dehydration for hunger.
- Staying hydrated supports detoxification processes and overall health during fasting.

- Use optimal hydration practices, including water, herbal teas, and electrolyte replenishment.
- With this essential guidance on nourishing your body during intermittent fasting, you can make informed dietary choices that align with your fasting goals.

As we conclude this chapter, remember that achieving success with intermittent fasting isn't solely a matter of understanding the physical aspects. The mental and emotional facets of your journey are equally crucial. Fasting is as much about the mind as it is about the body, so it's important that you find a balance that works best for you. In the next chapter, you'll discover how to create a sustainable fasting lifestyle that aligns with your personal goals and emotional well-being.

5

SUSTAINABLE FASTING: CRAFTING THE RIGHT MINDSET AND LIFESTYLE

You can think of intermittent fasting as an endurance challenge that requires you to have the right mindset and attain sustainability. In this chapter, you'll learn some myths about intermittent fasting, as well as how to make it a lifestyle, and finally some common beginner's mistakes. By the end of the chapter, you should be able to understand that intermittent fasting is a way of life and that you will make some mistakes along the way, but you must persevere in order to succeed.

DEBUNKING MYTHS

This eating approach has grown in popularity in recent years, and testimonies regarding its effectiveness in reducing weight continue to increase as more people use it. However, some people can't help but question the effectiveness of intermittent fasting, so it can be challenging to know if you should trust the successful stories or if the strategy is just hyped. You can choose for yourself after we address the myths that surround this way of life.

- **Intermittent fasting slows down metabolism.**

The truth: We looked at this in our opening chapter when listing some advantages of intermittent fasting. Intermittent fasting can actually increase metabolism by promoting fat loss and preserving lean muscle mass. While metabolism can slow down with age, intermittent fasting helps mitigate this effect.

- **Fasting leads to muscle loss.**

The truth: If you remember the list of benefits of intermittent fasting, you'll recall that it has proven to preserve and even increase lean muscle mass when combined with resistance training. Protein consumption during eating windows further supports muscle maintenance.

- **Intermittent fasting is unsafe for women over 50.**

The truth: Intermittent fasting is generally safe for a lot of people, including women over 50. We have discussed various health markers that intermittent fasting can improve already, making it a viable option. But remember that consultation with a healthcare provider is important for you in case you have a medical condition or you need help planning your diet.

- **Fasting causes hormonal imbalances in women.**

The truth: While fasting can affect hormones, it doesn't necessarily lead to imbalances. We have already talked about how intermittent fasting can improve insulin sensitivity and hormone regulation, which is beneficial for you, especially after going through menopausal changes.

- **Fasting makes you feel weak and worn out.**

The truth: Some initial fatigue can occur as your body adjusts to a new eating pattern. However, this is often temporary. With time, fasting may lead to increased energy levels and improved alertness.

- **Fasting causes nutritional deficiencies.**

The truth: As long as you do it right, intermittent fasting is not inherently linked to nutritional deficiencies. As you must know by now, intermittent fasting provides an opportunity to focus on nutrient-dense foods during your eating windows. This is because adopting a well-balanced diet is important for meeting your body's nutritional needs, and supplements can be used when necessary.

- **A lack of breakfast may contribute to increased weight gain.**

The truth: Contrary to popular assumption, skipping breakfast doesn't always result in gaining weight. According to controlled studies, between those who have breakfast and those who miss it, there is no difference in weight loss (Dhurandhar et al., 2014). Intermittent fasting simply condenses your daily eating window, but it's the quality of your food choices that matters most.

- **Weight loss results from fasting are guaranteed.**

The truth: While intermittent fasting can support weight loss, it's not a guarantee that anyone who starts it will automatically lose weight. Factors like the type of fasting method you chose, your food choices, and your overall calorie intake play a role. These factors contribute to how the impact of intermittent fasting on weight loss varies from person to person.

- **Weight loss is the only goal of fasting.**

The truth: Weight loss is one aspect of intermittent fasting, and we have already looked at the numerous other health benefits, which include improved metabolic health, improved immune system, and cardiovascular health to mention a few.

- **After age 50, it is too late to begin fasting.**

The truth: Age should not be a barrier to starting intermittent fasting. If anything, IF is effective for older adults, contributing to better health outcomes and quality of life.

I have shared with you the truth behind some misconceptions about intermittent fasting so you can feel more empowered and confident about the process. Now you know this approach is real, despite what some misinformed individuals may say.

TIPS FOR LONGEVITY

Your intermittent fasting approach has to be fun and enjoyable if you're in it for the long run. That way, you are less likely to get bored and quit. I know a friend who stopped after two months. Although she said she couldn't do it anymore because of the changes in her schedule when her grandchildren moved in, I realized that the problem was poor planning. You can live with people who eat regular meals and still fast—the key is in planning for longevity.

Making Intermittent Fasting a Permanent and Enjoyable Lifestyle

To make intermittent fasting a way of life, you need to do more than just stick to a certain eating schedule. You also need to create a habit that you enjoy and that helps you reach your long-term goals. In this section, we are now going to focus on how to make intermittent fasting a constant part of your life.

So, how can you continue with intermittent fasting even when it feels counterproductive to do so? Let's get right to it.

Holidays and Celebrations

These are the days of the calendar which are almost impossible to escape. If you know a holiday or special occasion is coming up, adjust your fasting schedule according to the time of activities. For example, if you will be having a family lunch date during a vacation, then you may want to set your fasting schedule in such a way that allows you to break your fast in time for that lunch date.

During festivities, use portion control to enjoy the foods you love in moderation. Do not get carried away by eating too much as a way of rewarding yourself for fasting. You want to be mindful when eating, after all. Also, don't get carried away with the fun and forget to drink plenty of water. Hydration can't be emphasized enough, and we have already covered its importance several times.

Social Events

Just like holidays, social events are unavoidable given that they are when you usually catch up and reconnect with the world. To improve your chances of sticking to intermittent fasting, let your friends and family know about your fasting routine. Most people will be understanding and supportive. When dining out or attending social gatherings, you'll also want to opt for healthier food options. Spoil yourself with salads, fresh fruits, lean proteins, and vegetables. Have you ever noticed how some people keep piling more food on their plates and wiping them clean during big events? Another important thing is to pay attention to your body's hunger cues and stop when you're satisfied. You don't have to finish everything on your plate, after all, so you can still watch your food intake during events.

Travel

If you are a traveler, you may be wondering about maintaining intermittent fasting while traveling long distances, for example, when you are on a long flight. The solution is easy—carry along nutritious snacks. Indeed, bring along your favorite foods, such as nuts, seeds, and dried fruits, to help you stay full on flights or other lengthy journeys. You will gain from adjusting to the new time zone as another improvement. If you're crossing time zones, gradually adjust your fasting schedule to match the local time.

Other Life Situations

You may find yourself in other situations than the ones we have discussed above, so it's crucial to prepare yourself for these as well.

It's important to put your health first, especially while you're sick. Don't hesitate to pause your fasting routine and focus on nourishing your body. If you are on medication, remember to consult your healthcare provider to ensure your fasting schedule doesn't interfere with their efficacy.

THE IMPORTANCE OF PERSONALIZATION

Personalization is the first step to making intermittent fasting a happy and healthy way of life. The strategy you choose for fasting should be based on your needs and circumstances. Here are some specific things you want to consider:

- **Picking the right method:** There are various intermittent fasting methods to choose from. Try out a few different ones to see which one works best with your plan and energy level. This could mean trying OMAD, TRE, or another method until you find the one that works best for you.
- **Fasting time:** Make the duration of fasting fit your schedule. Start your eating schedule early if you have more energy in the morning. If the evenings work better for you, make the necessary changes.
- **Adaptation period:** Allow your body some time to get used to the way you've chosen to fast. In the beginning, you may have some problems, but

these problems usually go away as your body gets used to the routine.

- **Health issues:** If you have specific health problems or worries, you should talk to a doctor or nurse. They can help you make changes to your fasting plan so that it works and is safe.

- **Society and lifestyle factors:** Intermittent fasting shouldn't get in the way of your daily life or relationships. You may tweak some things so that they fit in with your daily life. You can still eat with family and friends while following your fasting plan.

- **Occasional flexibility:** There's no problem with breaking your fasting plan once in a while. Unexpected things happen all the time, and adjusting as needed is the best way to keep fasting fun and stress-free.

- **State of mind:** Stay cheerful and think about how intermittent fasting will help you in the long run. Know that it's a journey and that it's normal to have failures or changes in your routine.

- **Keeping track of progress:** Monitoring your progress is an effective way to maintain your motivation. Keep an eye on your weight, energy level, happiness, and other health indicators to see how well intermittent fasting is working for you.

THE BENEFITS OF HAVING A FLEXIBLE INTERMITTENT FASTING SCHEDULE

One of the main reasons that make intermittent fasting great is that you can change the approach to fit your needs. It's not a set of strict rules, but a system that you can adjust to your convenience. Practicing intermittent fasting in a way that is both open and dedicated has many positive effects on your mind and emotions. This healthy way of thinking can help your health in these ways:

- **Reduced stress:** Being flexible lets you deal with life's unexpected turns without too much worry. You don't need to worry if a party or other important event goes outside of your fasting window. Lower stress levels are good for your mental health.
- **More fun:** You can enjoy meals with family and friends, taking advantage of the social and cultural parts of eating. In turn, this makes interactions stronger and makes eating more fun.
- **Freedom from guilt:** If you sometimes break your fasting plan, having a flexible attitude will keep you from feeling guilty. Everything is about balance, and being able to change your mind about what you eat can free you from feeling bad about it.
- **Sustainable commitment:** You're more likely to stick with intermittent fasting in the long run if

you can change your fasting schedule as needed. Over time, this dedication leads to better results.

- **Emotional resilience:** Being able to change how you do things helps you be emotionally resilient. Accepting changes and setbacks with grace is something that it teaches you. This can be good for your general emotional health.
- **Mindful eating:** Being flexible doesn't mean giving up being aware. In fact, it can encourage more mindful eating practices. When you do break your fast, you might appreciate your meals even more.
- **Empowerment:** Being open makes you feel like you have more control over your fasting schedule. This can make you feel better about your self-worth and improve your confidence.
- **Balance in your emotions:** Intermittent fasting can help keep your mood and emotions in check once you get used to it. Being flexible keeps you from getting too stuck on rules, which is good for your mental health.

Being flexible also helps you have a better relationship with food. It makes a point of saying that food is not the enemy and that eating should be fun.

ADDRESSING SLIP-UPS: HOW TO GET BACK ON TRACK WITHOUT GUILT

Mistakes and detours are natural parts of any journey, including this adventure you are on. You are more likely to make a lot of mistakes when trying out intermittent fasting for the first time. But where do you go after? How will you deal with the guilt?

When you feel guilty about making mistakes or not following your intermittent fasting plan, it can have a big effect on your mental health and slow you down in a number of ways, as we'll now discuss.

The Impact of Guilt and How It Hinders Your Progress

Guilt may cause you to feel bad about yourself. If you feel like you're failing or not following through with your fasting plan, the guilt can hurt your self-esteem and sense of worth, leading to a negative self-image. To prevent guilt from holding you back, you need to learn more about its impact.

- **Stress and anxiety:** Feeling guilty can make you anxious, which may interfere with your general emotional health. It can also make your body release stress hormones, which could create feelings of panic in your body.

- **Obsessive thoughts:** When you feel guilty, you might think too much about food, fasting, or your body. You may find that you can't stop thinking about what you ate or why you broke your fasting plan.
- **Disordered eating:** It's human nature to try and compensate for your guilt. Attempting to compensate for your perceived failures by restricting your food intake can be unhealthy and counterproductive. As time goes on, you may develop eating disorders like anorexia nervosa.
- **Fear of failure:** Feeling guilty all the time can make you afraid of failing, which may make you lose faith in your ability to stick to your fasting plan. This fear may cause you to hurt yourself over and over again.
- **Reduced enjoyment:** Feeling guilty makes you enjoy meals less. Instead, you may eat it with fear or worry and question yourself if you are doing it right.
- **Emotional roller coaster:** Experiencing guilt can turn your fasting journey into an emotional roller coaster. You might have moments of elation when you strictly adhere to your plan, followed by crashes of guilt when you deviate.
- **Inconsistent progress:** If guilt derails your fasting regimen, progress may become inconsistent. Instead of following a steady path toward your

goals, you may experience frequent stops and starts.

- **Burnout:** Prolonged guilt can lead to burnout. The emotional strain of constantly feeling guilty can exhaust your mental resources, potentially causing you to abandon your fasting routine altogether.
- **Impaired mindfulness:** Another effect of guilt is that it can distract you from mindful eating practices. You might not pay attention to the sensations of hunger and fullness, leading to overeating or undernourishing your body.

Dealing with your guilt is important for your mental health and the long-term success of intermittent fasting. It's important to know that making mistakes is normal and a part of the process. You can achieve a better, longer-lasting relationship with fasting and food if you learn how to handle these times without giving in to guilt.

How to Reframe From Slip-Ups

Here are some things you can do to turn mistakes into useful learning opportunities on your journey with intermittent fasting:

- **Practice self-compassion:** Instead of beating yourself up for not following your fasting schedule, treat yourself with the same compassion you would offer a friend who is in the same situation. Through self-compassion, your slip-ups will be viewed as opportunities of learning instead of failure.

- **Reflect and analyze:** Why did it happen? View the situation with a positive mindset and ask yourself: Did I have a tough day, an unexpected stress, or some sort of societal weight? You can then analyze it by noting down the triggers, so that next time, you are better prepared for it.
- **Set realistic expectations:** Remember, we are all humans, and intermittent fasting doesn't have to be rigid. Understand that minor variations do not define your entire fasting experience.
- **Focus on progress, not perfection:** It is uplifting to view progress from a perspective of progress rather than success or failure. Whenever you adhere to the plan, congratulate yourself because the occasional slip-up is just a minor glitch en route.
- **Avoid punitive measures:** Resist compensatory behaviors like fasting for too long or over-workout after making a blunder with your routine. Giving in to compensatory behaviors may create a vicious cycle.
- **Seek support and accountability:** Talk about it with someone you trust like friends, relatives, or a support group. You may find strength and encouragement in this simple act.

- **Track and learn:** Record your intermittent fasting experience in a journal. Recall the conditions that gave rise to careless slips and feelings you went through. With time, a pattern may be established which can enable you to anticipate and prevent any challenge that comes your way.
- **Plan for future challenges:** Learn from your mistakes and develop a plan to deal with such things in the future. Fasting could be effectively maintained through preparedness.
- **Celebrate small wins:** Give yourself credit and celebrate every little victory in your journey. These may include expanding your fasting window, avoiding unhealthy choices, and improving your ability to handle the pressures of life. These victories point out that you have made headway and survived.
- **Practice mindfulness and gratitude:** Be mindful when eating and appreciate what you are giving your body. This enhances your relationship with food and fasting.

MINDSET MATTERS: THE POWER OF POSITIVE THINKING

The connection between how you think and your ability to succeed with intermittent fasting, or any other change to your lifestyle, is a profound one. Your mindset, including your thoughts, beliefs, and attitudes, can have a big impact on your capacity to initiate and maintain fasting practices. The following is how you can reframe your mind and succeed in intermittent fasting:

- **Belief in your capability:** You're more likely to work hard and stick to your plan if you think you can do well with intermittent fasting. For you to be a moving force, you need to believe in your own abilities to deal with challenges and reach your goals.
- **Positive self-talk:** How you talk to yourself is important. You're more likely to stay inspired and on track if you talk to yourself in a positive and encouraging way every day. Talking badly to yourself can make you question your own abilities and fail at your goals.
- **Resilience in the face of challenges:** Having a good attitude helps you see problems as chances to grow instead of as things that you can't get past. This way, you're more likely to adapt, learn from mistakes, and keep going on your fasting journey.
- **Visualizing success:** You can achieve great results by first seeing yourself succeeding. If you are able to imagine yourself succeeding in reaching fasting objectives, the process of accomplishing them becomes more natural.
- **Embracing change:** Sometimes fasting means adjusting your eating behavior or routines. By viewing these as opportunities, a person with a

positive bent of mind adapts accordingly and easily navigates through the new changes.

- **Staying committed:** A positive mindset can help you stick to your goal even if there are great opportunities for temptation during your fasting period.
- **Dealing with stress:** Having a positive attitude can help you deal with stress better, which is important because stress and anxiety can make you eat too much or break your fasting plan.
- **Enjoy the journey:** Intermittent fasting shouldn't just be a way to get somewhere; it should be a way of life. Having a positive attitude can help you enjoy the process, which will make the trip last and be worth it.
- **Taking care of your health:** If you think positively, you may feel less stressed, have better mental health, and even be healthier physically. All of these things can help you fast more successfully.

You can cultivate positive thinking during intermittent fasting by having a mindset that promotes your capability for success, converting your challenges to opportunities, and making you more optimistic. You have the power to make intermittent fasting become a very powerful tool for creating a healthier and stronger life.

BEGINNER MISTAKES AND HOW TO AVOID THEM

Making blunders when beginning an intermittent fasting regimen is normal. Here are some typical mistakes that you may make, as well as some helpful advice and solutions to avoid them:

- **Overeating during eating windows:** This initial mistake is one way some people make up for fasting intervals. To avoid or solve this, always remember portion control whenever you eat. Try your best to pick nutrient-dense foods to satiate your appetite without consuming too many calories. Pay attention to your body's hunger signals and stop eating when you're full but not stuffed.
- **Ignoring hydration or electrolytes:** Not hydrating enough while fasting may result in dehydration. The solution for this is to drink water, herbal teas, or black coffee during the times you are fasting. You can also balance your electrolytes using electrolyte-enhanced water or homemade electrolyte drinks.
- **Having unrealistic fasting windows:** This means setting overly ambitious fasting windows that are hard to maintain. Consider starting with a smaller, more manageable fasting window and

gradually increase it. Start with 12 hours, for instance, then gradually increase to lengthier fasts.

- **A lack of planning:** Making impulsive food decisions is often a result of not making meals or fasting schedules in advance. To improve, try making a meal plan and setting some time for fasting. When it's time to eat, preparation ensures you have suitable, healthy selections available.

- **Rigid fasting regimens:** This is another common mistake that may lead to stress and fatigue when your regimen is overly strict. Be flexible with your fasting schedule. To accommodate social occasions, holidays, or days when your body requires a rest, adjust your timetable.

- **Skipping nutrient-rich foods:** Concentrating only on calorie intake without taking the nutritional value of the foods ingested into account is always a bad idea. Prioritize whole, nutrient-dense foods and ensure you get a variety of macronutrients and micronutrients for optimal health.

- **Skipping exercise:** When starting, you may avoid exercise during fasting, fearing energy depletion. Regular physical activity is beneficial during fasting. Consider starting with light exercises during fasting periods and gradually increasing intensity as you adjust.

- **Expecting quick results:** Unrealistic expectations can lead to disappointment. Keep in mind that intermittent fasting is not a magical diet that will make your problems disappear. Rather, it's a process you have to dedicate yourself to in order to reap its benefits. Realize that every person progresses differently. Instead of concentrating on rapid weight loss, try to also think of the long-term health advantages of intermittent fasting.

- **A lack of support:** Trying to manage intermittent fasting on your own, without assistance or direction, sometimes becomes lonely and may demoralize you. Try to find a fasting companion to share experiences with and ask for assistance when necessary, consult a healthcare professional, or join a community of people who are fasting.

- **Stressing over slip-ups:** This refers to allowing a feeling of guilt to cause little slip-ups that impede your growth. Accept mistakes as teaching moments. Take what you can from them and carry on with your fasting strategy without blaming yourself.

You can avoid potential pitfalls and enhance the success and sustainability of your intermittent fasting journey by recognizing and correcting these common beginner errors. Remember that change takes time, and that every step in the correct direction will improve your health and well-being.

KEY TAKEAWAYS

Debunking myths:

- Understand that many common myths surrounding intermittent fasting are unfounded and often contradicted by scientific evidence.
- Solidify your understanding of intermittent fasting's safety and efficacy through well-researched counterarguments.

Tips for longevity:

- Remember that flexibility and personalization are essential to make intermittent fasting a sustainable and enjoyable lifestyle.
- Learn how to adapt intermittent fasting to different life situations, ensuring it becomes a seamless part of your routine.

Addressing slip-ups:

- Acknowledge that slip-ups are normal and can be valuable learning experiences.
- Reframe mistakes positively, using them as stepping stones for growth rather than sources of guilt.

Mindset matters:

- Realize the serious influence of a positive, growth-oriented mindset on your intermittent fasting journey.
- Cultivate this mindset through actionable strategies, like affirmations and visualization.

Beginner mistakes and how to avoid them:

- Learn about common pitfalls and how to steer clear of them, such as overeating after a fast.
- Embrace the power of patience and continual learning, adapting to your unique needs.

Internalizing these takeaways equips you to practice intermittent fasting with confidence and resilience. Your mindset and approach play a significant role in your success on this journey.

As we come to the end of this chapter, it's important to remember that having holistic well-being is about more than diet and mindset alone; exercise is also very important. Intermittent fasting, a good attitude, and the right kind of exercise can change your life.

In the next chapter, we'll go into more detail about exercise, with a focus on what women over 50 need. You'll learn how to use the power of intermittent fasting along with exercise to reach your full potential and live a healthy, happy life. Get ready to start this energizing trip as we explore fitness in a way that is just right for you.

6

LET'S GET MOVING

Another common myth about intermittent fasting is that working out while fasting is harmful or dangerous. However, studies have shown that intermittent fasting coupled with exercise has positive effects on weight loss and metabolic health (Vieira et al., 2016).

Here is a real-life story to demonstrate the positive impact of intermittent fasting when paired with exercise. It's an inspiring story about a woman we'll call Gina. When Gina was 63, she decided to work on improving her health upon retiring. She used to weigh 287 pounds but lost 80 pounds in eight months through walking and intermittent fasting. Now, she weighs 207 pounds and is aiming for 180. Isn't that amazing?

Gina acknowledges that her diet isn't the healthiest because she prefers pizza and hamburgers over salads. However, she tracks her exercise and food intake, ensuring she stays away from junk food and sweets when she's home and tries to consume no more than 1,500 calories most days. She fasts for 13 hours every night and also stays hydrated with 101 ounces of water daily, which is a crucial part of her routine.

Before Gina retired, she would barely walk 6,000 steps in a day, so she knew that she needed to make some changes in her life. After retiring, she set a goal of walking 10,000 steps a day and often surpasses 12,000 now. She combines walking with weightlifting at the gym and bowling during the fall and winter. Her story shows how commitment to exercise and intermittent fasting can lead to a healthier and more active lifestyle.

MENOPAUSE AND EXERCISE

Do you remember the changes we discussed in the first chapter during menopause and the immediate post-menopausal phase? If not, let me help you recall. During and after menopause, your body undergoes significant physiological changes, including a decline in estrogen levels, which may lead to various changes like weight gain, mood swings, and hot flashes. These changes can be challenging, but exercise helps alleviate many of these symptoms, which brings us to some of its benefits below:

- **Improves weight management:** It's common for some women to gain weight during menopause because of changes in hormones, especially around the abdomen. But that should never make you lose hope, as working out regularly improves your metabolism and burns calories, which makes it easier to keep off weight or lose it.
- **Regulates your mood:** Mood swings, anger, and even signs of depression or worry can happen during menopause. Studies show that when you exercise, your body releases endorphins, which are natural chemicals that make you feel good. Exercise also reduces stress and anxiety by triggering the release of neurotransmitters like serotonin and dopamine (Collins, 2012). This might help you feel happier and more emotionally stable.
- **Reduces hot flashes:** Even though exercise may not immediately prevent hot flashes, it lessens both their frequency and intensity. Regular exercise regulates body temperature, reducing the severity of hot flashes. In fact, a study reveals that menopausal women who exercised saw a 60% decrease in the frequency of their hot flashes (MGH Center for Women's Mental Health, 2017).
- **Improves bone health:** Because of the decreased estrogen levels, menopausal women are more susceptible to osteoporosis. Studies show that weight-bearing exercises in postmenopausal

women like walking, running, and weight lifting may help maintain bone strength and density, and lower the risk of fractures (Zehnacker & Bemis-Dougherty, 2007).

- **Promotes heart and vascular health:** The loss of estrogen during menopause is linked to an increase in heart disease risk factors (Anagnostis et al., 2022). Regular exercise is good for your heart because it lowers bad cholesterol, raises good cholesterol, and improves general heart function.
- **Aids in better sleep:** During menopause, many women have trouble sleeping or suffer from outright insomnia. Exercise helps you sleep better by balancing circadian rhythms and easing the signs of insomnia.

Remember that the type of exercise you do and how hard you work out should depend on your health and fitness level. Intermittent fasting and exercise can be good for most people, but it might not be right for everyone. It's important to talk to a healthcare provider who will factor in your personal health, the level of exercise you put in, and your nutritional needs.

Low Impact Workouts

These are perfect exercise options if you have joint pain, injuries, or if you want a gentle massage. This is because the movements in these routines are usually not very intense nor do they require you to use a lot of force.

Here is why these exercises are advantageous especially during and after menopause:

- **Joint-friendly:** Low-impact workouts are friendly to the joints and are recommended for females who may suffer from arthritis, joint pain, or a history of joint problems (CDC, 2022). They lessen the chance of the spine, hips, and knees suffering from excessive wear and strain.
- **Bone health:** Walking, swimming, or utilizing elliptical machines are examples of low-impact exercises that nonetheless support bone density and strength without having the same jarring effects as high-impact exercises like running or jumping.
- **Cardiovascular health:** Low-impact exercises can effectively condition the heart, aid in weight control, and lower the chance of developing heart disease. They do this without the intense pounding on the heart and arteries which is common in high-impact exercises.
- **Injury prevention:** We have already talked about how we may be more vulnerable to harm as we age due to physiological changes. Low-impact exercises assist in increasing flexibility, stability,

and balance, which lowers the likelihood of falling and the resulting injuries.

- **Sustainability:** These exercises are less demanding for most individuals of all fitness levels and ages, which makes them easier to maintain. They are safe to do over and over again without getting hurt or burned out, so they are good for long-term health and fitness upkeep.
- **Comfort and pleasure:** These exercises are more pleasant and appealing for many women. Low-impact workouts are a great way to improve your heart health, muscle strength, and flexibility without putting too much stress on your body.

Forms of Low-Impact Workouts

Examples of low-impact exercises vary, including even sitting! If you have problems with mobility, seated exercises can work out best for you. You can do these in a chair and focus on light movements, such as leg lifts, seated marches, and seated leg extensions.

Here are more low-impact exercises:

- **Walking:** Surprised? Walking is a great low-impact workout that can be done anywhere and at any tempo, making it convenient for all fitness levels. A daily brisk walk can improve your cardiovascular health, weight, and leg strength.

- **Resistance band exercises:** Resistance bands increase muscle strength and do not require a lot of force. They work for leg lifts, shoulder presses, and bicep curls.
- **Swimming:** While it's a relaxing hobby, swimming helps reduce stress on joints while providing a full-body workout, helping you with strength and flexibility.
- **Cycling:** Cycling targets lower body muscles, whether you are using a stationary bike or a real one outdoors. As a result, you will strengthen your legs and improve heart health while minimizing joint stress.
- **Yoga:** You probably know yoga for its flexibility, balance, and relaxation. This improves muscular tone and joint mobility best. In addition, yoga reduces stress and improves mental wellness.
- **Pilates:** Pilates focuses on building core strength, flexibility, and understanding the body as a whole. It works especially well for toning and building the muscles in your back and abdomen. Pilates movements can be adjusted to match your fitness level.
- **Tai chi:** Tai chi is a graceful martial art that's recognized for enhancing balance, coordination, and fall prevention.
- **Elliptical exercises:** A gym elliptical can substitute running or jogging. With this, it will

help work out your upper and lower muscles, making it a full-body workout.

- **Balance and flexibility exercises:** Standing on one foot, light stretching, and simple balance postures can help reduce falls.

How to Fit Low-Impact Exercises in Your Daily Life

The following are suggestions you can follow to incorporate low-impact exercises into your daily activities:

- **Morning stretch:** To warm up your muscles and make you more flexible, start your day with a 15-minute stretching exercise.
- **Active commuting:** If you take public transportation, you might want to get off at an earlier stop and walk the rest of the way to your location.
- **Activity-based transportation:** For short trips to the store, your workplace, or for nearby errands, walk or ride a bike instead of driving. This will make you more active and lower your carbon footprint at the same time.
- **The stair challenge:** Try taking the stairs instead of the elevator whenever you can. Taking the stairs is a great way to strengthen your lower body and do some cardio.
- **Exercise errands:** Make physical exercise a part of your daily tasks. You can walk between stores

or use a shopping cart to add some light resistance to your shopping trips if you plan them well.

- **Workout partner:** You can also find a coworker or friend who likes working out as much as you do. Working out with a friend can keep you inspired and make it more fun. You and your friend can go for walks during lunch or work out together before or after work.
- **Making the most of your free time:** Do something active in your free time, like dancing, yoga, stretching, or walks. To get more energy, take breaks at work to stretch, walk around the office, or do some movements in your chair.
- **Workouts at your desk:** Do exercises like seated leg lifts, ankle circles, and shoulder rolls at your desk without drawing attention to yourself to keep your body moving during long work hours.
- **Short workouts:** When you get a chance, do a short workout during the day, like yoga stretches or 5-minute bodyweight movements.
- **Family activity:** Get your family to do healthy activities with you. Plan walks or bike rides with them or play active games together.
- **Lawn care:** Gardening can sometimes be good for your body. You may get some exercise and enjoy the outdoors by digging, pulling weeds, and sowing seeds.

- **Breaks for dancing:** Play your favorite music and dance whenever you feel like it during the day. It's fun to dance, and it can also make you feel better.

STRENGTH TRAINING

Resistance training, which is another name for strength training, is a type of exercise that builds muscle strength and stamina. For this kind of exercise, you work against resistance, which can come from tools, free weights, resistance bands, or even your own body weight. To create a good fitness program, you'll need to include strength training because the exercises help build strength and muscle.

Let's look into how strength training can help both peri and postmenopausal women:

- **Prevention of osteoporosis:** Weight-bearing activities, such as strength training, put stress and tension on the bones. Mechanical loading encourages bone cells to make more bone tissue, as a result increasing bone density and lowering the risk of osteoporosis, a disorder that causes brittle and frail bones.
- **Rebuilding muscle mass:** We looked at how muscle mass is lost as you get older, affecting your strength and mobility. The good news is that strength training supports functional

independence in daily activities by rebuilding and maintaining muscle mass.

- **Blood pressure control:** It has been demonstrated that regular strength training lowers resting blood pressure, which may help to improve cardiovascular health (Westcott, 2012).
- **Improved blood lipid profiles:** Engaging in resistance training can lead to favorable changes in blood lipid profiles by increasing good cholesterol and reducing bad cholesterol and triglycerides.
- **Blood sugar control:** Strength training helps the body's insulin sensitivity, making it more efficient at using blood sugar. This can be especially important for managing blood sugar levels, reducing the risk of type 2 diabetes, and addressing blood sugar fluctuations common during menopause.
- **Enhanced physical performance:** Strength training can increase your physical performance, making daily chores easier to handle and more enjoyable.
- **Cancer risk reduction:** While no one lifestyle can ensure total immunity from diseases like cancer, there is evidence to suggest that regular strength training may help lower the risk of some cancers (National Cancer Institute, 2020).

Beginner-Friendly Strength Training Exercises

You may be wondering which strength training exercise to start with. Below is a list of some friendly strength training exercises to get you started. It's wise to start with light weights, then gradually increase the resistance as you become more comfortable.

Bodyweight squats:

- With your feet standing at shoulder-width apart, initiate the descent by gradually bending your knees and shifting your hips backward.
- Maintain an upright posture with your back straight and chest elevated.
- Propel yourself back to the initial standing position by exerting force through your heels.

Wall push-ups:

- Stand facing a wall and move your feet a few strides backward.
- With your hands aligned with your shoulders on the wall, push your chest toward the wall by bending your elbows.
- Push away from the wall to return to your original stance.

Dumbbell bicep curls:

- Grasp a dumbbell in each hand, and extend your arms out by your sides.
- Lift the dumbbells in the direction of your shoulders by flexing your elbows.
- Lower the dumbbells to their initial position.

Dumbbell rows:

- Hold a dumbbell in your right hand and position your left knee and hand on a bench.
- Ensure that your back remains parallel to the ground.
- Draw the dumbbell toward your hip, maintaining your elbow's proximity to your body.
- Return your right hand to the starting position and repeat for both sides.

Chair dips:

- Using a sturdy chair, sit on the edge with your hands holding onto its front edge.
- Shift your feet forward, elevating your buttocks off the chair.
- Lower your body down by bending your elbows.
- Push with your palms to restore yourself to the initial position.

Leg raises:

- Put your arms at your sides and lie on your back.
- Elevate your legs from the ground while keeping them fully extended.
- Lower your legs, allowing them to hover just above the ground.
- Repeat this movement without allowing your feet to make contact with the ground.

Planks:

- Assume a push-up position, resting on your forearms with your elbows bent at 90 degrees and your weight evenly distributed.
- Maintain a straight alignment from your head to your heels.
- Sustain this position for as long as possible, with the goal of extending your duration in subsequent sessions.

Remember to warm up before your strength training routine and cool down afterward. You can start with 1 to 2 sets of 10 to 12 repetitions for each exercise, then gradually progress by adding more sets or repetitions as you become more comfortable. Listen to your body, and if you have any existing health concerns, consult with a healthcare provider or fitness professional before beginning a new exercise program.

FINDING YOUR FIT

Exercise must, of course, be tailored to your goals and needs. Because of this, your exercise routine will be different from that of another person. Below are some points to consider when choosing the right fit:

- **Check your current fitness level:** Consider your strength, stamina, ability to adapt, and balance. Having an idea of these things gives you a starting point. You can put yourself to the test with some simple exercises, such as walking at a certain speed for a set amount of time or doing as many bodyweight squats as you can in five minutes. From there, you will be able to determine how much exercise you may start with.
- **Make clear goals:** Write down some goals for your workout. How you work out depends on what you want to achieve. For example, when you want to lose weight, your main goal is to do aerobic exercises like cycling or fast walks, but if you want to build muscles, then strength training is what you need.
- **Take into account any injuries or health problems:** Talk to a doctor, and a physical trainer too, if you have any preexisting injuries or health concerns. They may assist you with finding the right exercises for you. For example, if you have

knee problems, you might be recommended to try activities like swimming or riding a bike.

- **Don't forget your experience:** How much exercise you've done before also matters. If you are just starting out, you may start with easy workouts like brisk walks or bodyweight exercises. After getting the hang of it, more workout routines can be added. If you have more experience, you might do more intense exercises, such as band resistance or lifting some dumbbells.

- **Take your body type into account:** What exercises you enjoy or are best suited for you may depend on physical factors like your body shape. In this instance, an ectomorph can concentrate on performing more strength training exercises to build muscle, whereas an endomorph can concentrate on doing more cardiovascular workouts to manage weight.

TIPS FOR CREATING A BALANCED EXERCISE ROUTINE

Creating a balanced workout routine is important because it ensures that all muscle groups are targeted and developed evenly. This helps prevent muscle imbalances and reduces the risk of injury. A balanced workout routine also allows for proper recovery and prevents boredom, which improves overall fitness and well-being.

Here are some tips for incorporating various elements into your routine:

- **Set realistic goals:** Your goals guide you when selecting exercises and tracking progress, so they should be clear and realistic.
- **Warm-up and cool down:** Prior to exercise, warm up with light cardio and dynamic stretches. Afterward, cool down with static stretches to prevent muscle stiffness.
- **Do cardiovascular exercises:** A good starting point is a weekly target of 150 minutes of moderate-intensity aerobic activity. To switch things up, consider having short bursts of intense exercise followed by brief rest periods.
- **Engage in strength training:** When starting, two days a week is a good target for training exercises. For these days, you can involve bodyweight exercises, free weights, resistance bands, or weight machines. Focus on working all major muscle groups, including the chest, back, legs, and core.
- **Do some flexibility training:** Dedicate time to flexibility training to improve your range of motion and to prevent injuries. Pilates and yoga are excellent options. You can perform stretching exercises daily or as part of your workout routine.
- **Consider your balance and stability:** As you age, balance and stability exercises become crucial.

Activities such as tai chi can help improve balance and reduce the risk of falls.

- **Stay hydrated and eat well:** Proper hydration and nutrition are essential for fueling your workouts and aiding recovery. Ensure you stay hydrated and consume a balanced diet.

- **Rest and recover:** Don't forget the importance of rest and recovery. Allow your body time to heal between workouts to prevent overuse injuries. Try to get adequate sleep to support recovery and overall well-being.

- **Vary your routine:** Try to incorporate variety into your workouts because changing exercises keeps things interesting while helping prevent overuse injuries. Explore different forms of exercise, like dancing, hiking, or recreational sports, to keep things fresh.

- **Listen to your body:** Pay attention to how your body responds to exercise. If you experience pain or discomfort, adjust your routine accordingly. If you have any medical conditions or are taking medications, consult your healthcare provider for exercise recommendations.

- **Stay consistent:** Try to stick to a regular exercise schedule to see long-term benefits. It's better to exercise moderately but consistently than sporadically.

- **Track your progress:** Consider keeping a workout journal or using fitness apps to track your progress and set new goals as you achieve milestones. Keep in mind that each person requires a different amount of exercise. Make sure your regimen contains the essential components of cardiovascular, strength, and flexibility training while also being tailored to your particular goals and preferences.

STAYING MOTIVATED

Motivation is important in ensuring you remain committed to exercising consistently. In this section, we'll discuss the importance of motivation and some strategies to help you stay pumped up.

Consistency is one of the benefits of staying motivated. The greatest benefits come from regular exercise. Motivation keeps you from missing any of your workout sessions. This means the higher your motivation, the more you work out, and the greater the positive impact on your well-being, so exercise is worth the time and effort.

Motivation ensures that you monitor your progress as well as work toward your fitness goals. Keeping your motivation also makes exercising a habit and a normal routine that becomes a part of your lifestyle with time.

Strategies to Stay Motivated

- **Set clear goals:** Set clear, attainable exercise goals. Setting goals keeps you going, whether you want to lose weight, get stronger, or increase your fitness.
- **Find enjoyable activities:** Make sure to select activities that you really enjoy so that you can always look forward to exercising.
- **Change your routine:** To keep things interesting, switch up your workouts. To keep things interesting and new, try out new sports, workouts, or lessons.
- **Create a schedule:** Ensure that you create a regular exercise schedule, which will motivate you to work toward a common goal.
- **Work out with a friend:** Make a regular time to work out. Being consistent makes it easy to stay motivated because it turns into a habit.
- **Track your progress:** Look at your progress to see how far you've come. This can inspire you and help you make the changes you need to make to your habit.
- **Reward yourself:** Don't hesitate to treat yourself to your favorite meal or spend a day to yourself as a reward for doing well.
- **Visualize success:** Picture the good things that will happen because of your fitness practice, like

being healthier, having more energy, or feeling better about your own self-confidence.

- **Join a fitness community:** Take part in workout groups or classes. A feeling of belonging to a group can motivate and inspire you.
- **Use technology:** It's become easy to set reminders and keep track of your progress using fitness apps and wearable devices such as smartwatches.
- **Set mini-goals:** Break larger goals into smaller, more achievable objectives. Celebrate these mini-goals along the way.
- **Stay informed:** Learn about the benefits of various exercises, the latest fitness trends, and the science behind them. Knowledge can be motivating.
- **Accept setbacks:** Understand that setbacks happen. They're just part of the trip. Don't be discouraged by them. Instead, use these experiences to learn new things.
- **Find inspiration:** Read success stories and watch motivating videos of other people, or simply follow fitness influencers as an inspiration for your workout.
- **Take accountability:** Share your goals with someone reliable who will ensure you are accountable.

You should also realize that your motivation may change over time. When it's low, work on being disciplined and making new habits. And when it's high, use that energy to move forward on your exercise path. In the end, keeping your motivation going is an ongoing process. The most important thing is to figure out what works best for you.

KEY TAKEAWAYS

Menopause and exercise:

- Exercise alleviates common symptoms of menopause, such as weight gain, mood swings, and hot flashes.
- It also helps prevent conditions like osteoporosis and improves overall health during this life stage.

Low-impact workouts:

- Examples include walking, swimming, and Pilates, which provide excellent cardiovascular and muscular benefits.
- These exercises are ideal in and beyond your 50s because they are gentle on the joints.

Strength training:

- Strength training offers numerous benefits, including preventing osteoporosis, building muscle mass, and improving cardiovascular health.

- It's especially vital for women over 50 to maintain physical performance and combat various health conditions.

Finding your fit:

- Assessing your fitness level and setting clear goals is essential for creating an effective workout plan.
- You are not in this for a one-size-fits-all solution; your exercise routine should align with your goals, body type, experience, and any health conditions.

Staying motivated:

- Strategies such as setting goals, varying your routine, tracking progress, and seeking social support can help you stay on track, which is crucial for a consistent workout plan.

These key takeaways emphasize the importance of exercise, tailored to individual needs, to improve health and well-being. Staying motivated and finding the right fitness approach can lead to a more fulfilling and sustainable fitness journey.

7

SUPPORTING YOUR INTERMITTENT FASTING JOURNEY

 Let food be thy medicine, and medicine be thy food.

— HIPPOCRATES

As you venture into intermittent fasting, the quality of your nutrition becomes the foundation of your success. Your experience is influenced by the time of day you eat, as well as the sort of food you eat. In this chapter, we will explore some practical strategies to support your intermittent fasting lifestyle by eating nutritious foods, preparing strategically, and learning the usefulness of keeping track of what you eat.

MEAL PLANNING 101

Meal planning is crucial when practicing intermittent fasting because it helps ensure that you consume balanced and nutritious meals during your eating window. It allows you to make conscious choices about the types of foods you eat, helping you maintain a healthy and sustainable eating pattern. Planning meals also helps prevent impulsive food choices or overeating because you will have preplanned meals ready to go.

How to Create a Balanced Meal Plan

When you're new to intermittent fasting, planning your meals may seem like a challenge, so here are some steps to help you master them.

- **Step 1: Understand your intermittent fasting window.**

Your intermittent fasting window determines the structure of your meal plan. If you're following the 16:8 method, your daily eating window is eight hours, while 5:2 might require specific fasting days. It's important to take note of your specific schedule so that you can make a meal plan that works for you.

- **Step 2: Prioritize nutrient density.**

This can not be emphasized enough—add foods that are high in nutrients to your meals. These are full of minerals, vitamins, and other important nutrients that women over 50 need the most. Fruits, veggies, lean proteins, and whole grains are some examples. Not only do these foods keep you full during fasting times, they also help your body stay healthy.

- **Step 3: Balance your macronutrients.**

When planning your meals, try to balance the macronutrients which are proteins, carbohydrates, and healthy fats. Proteins help with muscle repair and maintenance, while carbohydrates offer immediate energy. Healthy fats support hormonal balance and keep you satisfied. A general meal plan should reflect this balance well.

- **Step 4: Remember portion control and caloric awareness**

While intermittent fasting isn't primarily about calorie counting, it's essential to maintain a rough awareness of your daily intake. Monitor your portions, ensuring they match your goals, whether it's weight loss, maintenance, or muscle building.

- **Step 5: Hydrate.**

Remember how important it is to stay hydrated when you are eating or when you are fasting. Staying hydrated is good for your health and nutrition. Fruits like watermelons are high in water, so it can be a good idea to add them to your diet to stay hydrated.

Meal planning guarantees that your body is receiving the proper nutrients and it also promotes your general well-being. You'll be better prepared to make meal plans that are specific to your intermittent fasting schedule and objectives if you keep these steps in mind.

Practical Tips for Weekly Meal Plan

You can't always plan your meal every day, so for convenience's sake, it's best to plan your meals weekly. This will provide a clear road map and prepare you mentally for what lies ahead. Here are some tips on how to make weekly meal plans:

- **Plan your menu:** Begin by creating a weekly menu. This should be in line with your intermittent fasting schedule and balance your nutrients.
- **Make a grocery list:** Once your menu is ready, draft a detailed grocery list. This list will help you shop efficiently and ensure you have all the

necessary ingredients on hand. It can also prevent impulsive purchases that might not align with your meal plan.

- **Choose a prep day:** Select a day of the week for your meal prep session. Many people find that Sunday works well, as it sets them up for the week ahead. However, pick a day that is suitable for you.

- **Consider getting meal prep containers:** You can step up your meal planning game with good-quality meal prep containers. Pick different sizes to accommodate different dishes. These containers will not only keep your meals fresh but also help with portion control.

- **Portion your meals:** When packing your meals, portion them into your meal prep containers. To avoid overeating or wasting food, ensure your portion sizes align with your daily calorie intake.

- **Prepare in batches:** Cook in batches to save time. For instance, you can prepare a large pot of soup, a batch of roasted vegetables, or a quantity of grains like quinoa or brown rice. This way, you'll have versatile ingredients ready to assemble into meals on different days.

- **Mix and match components:** Plan meals with interchangeable components. For example, prepare a protein source (like grilled chicken or tofu), a variety of veggies, and a whole grain (like quinoa). Then, pair these components with different companions to enjoy a variety of meals throughout the week.

- **Label and date:** Don't forget to label your containers with the contents and date. This way, you can be sure you're eating fresh food and also avoid food wastage by consuming packed food before it goes bad.
- **Stay creative:** Variety is key to maintaining your enthusiasm for meal prep. Experiment with different recipes and flavor profiles to keep your meals exciting.
- **Be consistent:** Consistency is the key to successful meal prepping. Once you establish a routine, it becomes a seamless part of your weekly schedule.

You'll save time and lessen the stress of meal preparation throughout your fasting and eating windows if you learn the art of meal preparation. It's a realistic and efficient method to assist your intermittent fasting experience while making sure you always have nourishing and tasty food on hand.

7-DAY MEAL PLANS

Taking into account the three intermittent fasting methods we discussed in Chapter 3, here are some flexible plans that you can adjust to suit your preferences.

Time-Restricted Eating: 16:8 Meal Plan

Day 1: Eating window: 12:00 p.m. to 8:00 p.m.

- **Lunch:** Grilled chicken breast with quinoa and roasted vegetables
- **Snack:** Greek yogurt with fresh fruit
- **Dinner:** Steamed broccoli with baked salmon and brown rice

Day 2: Eating window: 12:00 p.m. to 8:00 p.m.

- **Lunch:** Lentil soup with a side salad
- **Snack:** Sliced cucumbers with hummus
- **Dinner:** Mixed vegetables with stir-fried tofu and brown rice

Day 3: Eating window: 12:00 p.m. to 8:00 p.m.

- **Lunch:** Turkey and avocado wrap with whole-grain tortilla
- **Snack:** Apple chips
- **Dinner:** Steamed asparagus and grilled shrimp with cauliflower rice

Day 4: Eating window: 11:30 a.m. to 7:30 p.m.

- **Lunch:** Spinach and feta omelet with a side of whole-grain toast

- **Snack:** Carrot and celery sticks with hummus
- **Dinner:** Baked chicken with sweet potatoes and green beans

Day 5: Eating window:12:00 p.m. to 8:00 p.m.

- **Lunch:** Quinoa salad with chickpeas, tomatoes, and cucumbers
- **Snack:** Greek yogurt with honey
- **Dinner:** Beef stir-fry with broccoli and brown rice

Day 6: Eating window: 11:30 a.m. to 7:30 p.m.

- **Lunch:** Caprese salad with mozzarella, tomatoes, and basil
- **Snack:** Chocolate and mixed nuts
- **Dinner:** Chickpea salad and grilled tuna with zucchini noodles

Day 7: Eating window: 12:00 p.m. to 8:00 p.m.

- **Lunch:** Avocado salad and fried rice
- **Snack:** Sliced apples with almond butter
- **Dinner:** Baked turkey with sweet potatoes and green beans

Time-Restricted Eating: 18:6 Meal Plan

Day 1: Eating window: 9:00 a.m. to 3:00 p.m.

- **Breakfast:** Greek yogurt with honey and mixed berries
- **Lunch:** Quinoa salad with grilled chicken and mixed vegetables

Day 2: Eating window: 10:30 a.m. to 4:30 p.m.

- **Breakfast:** Scrambled eggs with spinach and feta
- **Lunch:** Lentil soup with a side salad

Day 3: Eating window: 9:00 a.m. to 3:00 p.m.

- **Breakfast:** Simple banana oatmeal with almond butter
- **Lunch:** Fried asparagus and grilled salmon with cauliflower rice

Day 4: Eating window: 10:30 a.m. to 4:30 p.m.

- **Breakfast:** Whole-grain toast with avocado and poached eggs
- **Lunch:** Steamed broccoli and fried brown rice with tofu stir-fry

Day 5: Eating window: 9:00 a.m. to 3:00 p.m.

- **Breakfast:** Pineapple cubes and a glass of milk
- **Lunch:** Avocado wrap and grilled turkey

Day 6: Eating window: 10:30 a.m. to 4:30 p.m.

- **Breakfast:** Smoothie with spinach, banana, and protein powder
- **Lunch:** Quinoa salad with chickpeas, tomatoes, and cucumbers

Day 7: Eating window: 9:00 a.m. to 3:00 p.m.

- **Breakfast:** Mixed fruit salad with a drizzle of honey
- **Lunch:** Grilled chicken breast with sweet potatoes and green beans

7-Day Meal Plan for One Meal a Day

Day 1: Meal window: 6:00 p.m. to 7:00 p.m.

- **Meal:** Grilled salmon with quinoa, steamed broccoli, and a mixed greens salad

Day 2: Meal window: 6:30 p.m. to 7:30 p.m.

- **Meal:** Mixed vegetables with stir-fried tofu and brown rice
- **Dessert:** 2 bars dark chocolate

Day 3: Meal window: 6:15 p.m. to 7:15 p.m.

- **Meal:** Baked chicken with sweet potatoes, asparagus, and a side of sautéed spinach

Day 4: Meal window: 6:45 p.m. to 7:45 p.m.

- **Meal:** Roasted brussels sprouts and quinoa with beef stir-fry
- **Dessert:** A piece of fruit

Day 5: Meal window: 6:10 p.m. to 7:10 p.m.

- **Meal:** Lentil soup with a side salad and a whole-grain roll.

Day 6: Meal window: 6:40 p.m. to 7:40 p.m.

- **Meal:** Grilled shrimp with brown rice, grilled zucchini, and a side of hummus with carrot sticks

Day 7: Meal window: 6:20 p.m. to 7:20 p.m.

- **Meal:** Green tuna salad with a balsamic vinaigrette dressing

Conclude the week with a small serving of yogurt with honey.

7-Day Meal Plan for 5:2 Intermittent Diet

Day 1 (Fasting day)

- **Breakfast:** Ginger tea with mint and lemon
- **Lunch:** Plain vegetable broth
- **Dinner:** Grilled skinless chicken breast with steamed broccoli and a squeeze of lemon with a small portion of brown rice or quinoa

Day 2 (Non-fasting day)

- **Breakfast:** Whole-grain toast, scrambled eggs with spinach, and cherry tomatoes
- **Lunch:** Quinoa and vegetable salad with a lemon-tahini dressing
- **Snack:** Fresh fruit
- **Dinner:** Baked salmon with a side of roasted sweet potatoes and asparagus

Day 3 (Fasting day)

- **Breakfast:** Plain chicken soup
- **Lunch:** Lemon tea with a bit of honey
- **Dinner:** Mixed greens salad with a variety of colorful vegetables

Day 4 (Non-fasting day)

- **Breakfast:** Greek yogurt with honey and mixed berries
- **Lunch:** A whole-grain wrap with lean turkey, mixed greens, and a touch of hummus
- **Snack:** A handful of mixed nuts
- **Dinner:** Stir-fried tofu with brown rice and vegetable greens

Day 5 (Non-Fasting day)

- **Breakfast:** Spinach omelet with diced carrots
- **Lunch:** Baked sweet potatoes with vegetable salad
- **Snack:** Whole grain crackers
- **Dinner:** Grilled chicken breast with a side of steamed green beans, and a small portion of quinoa

Day 6 (Non-fasting day)

- **Breakfast:** Simple banana oatmeal with some honey
- **Lunch:** Mixed greens salad with grilled shrimp and a light vinaigrette
- **Snack:** A piece of fruit
- **Dinner:** Baked cod with roasted butternut squash and sautéed spinach

Day 7 (Non-fasting day)

- **Breakfast:** Sautéed mushrooms with scrambled eggs and a whole-grain English muffin
- **Lunch:** Black bean salad and cauliflower rice
- **Snack:** Greek yogurt with a sprinkle of nuts
- **Dinner:** Grilled lean steak with a side of quinoa and grilled zucchini

With the flexible meal plans above, you can swap some meals for your healthy favorites without messing up your intermittent fasting journey. You can also experiment with new recipes so the fun doesn't run out.

RECIPE IDEAS: NUTRIENT-RICH DISHES TO FUEL YOUR FASTING BODY

It's easy to fast well and still eat healthily. Here are some nutrient-rich recipes that are best for post-fast meals. The recipes also work well if you prefer vegetarian or gluten-free options because they leave room for such dietary preferences.

Protein-Packed Quinoa Salad

This is a high-protein and fiber-rich salad to refuel your body after a fast.

Time: 41 minutes

Servings: 3

Nutritional information:

Calories	409
Carbs	43.8 grams
Protein	25.6 grams
Fat	15 grams

Ingredients:

- 1 cup quinoa
- 2 cups water
- 8 oz grilled chicken breast, diced (or 1 can of chickpeas for a vegetarian option)

- 1 cup cherry tomatoes, halved
- 1 cucumber, diced
- ¼ cup red onion, finely chopped
- ¼ cup fresh parsley, chopped
- 2 tbsp olive oil
- 2 tbsp lemon juice
- ⅛ tsp salt
- ⅛ tsp pepper

Directions:

1. Rinse the quinoa under cold water. In a saucepan, bring 2 cups of water to a boil, then add quinoa, then lower the heat.
2. Cover and leave to simmer for about 16 minutes. Let the quinoa cool once it becomes tender.
3. In a large bowl, combine the cooked quinoa, grilled chicken or chickpeas, cherry tomatoes, cucumber, red onion, and fresh parsley.
4. Use a small bowl to combine the salt, lemon juice, olive oil, and pepper. Whisk well, then drizzle it over the quinoa salad and mix it in.
5. Chill the salad for at least 30 minutes before serving.

Special notes:

You can improve the salad with your favorite veggies or add a sprinkle of feta cheese for extra flavor. The protein content makes this recipe a good option for a post-workout meal.

Vegan Avocado and Black Bean Tacos

A plant-based, gluten-free option packed with healthy fats and fiber.

Time: 4 minutes

Servings: 4

Nutritional information:

Calories	376
Carbs	43.8 grams
Protein	7.6 grams
Fat	19.7 grams

Ingredients:

- 2 tbsp lime juice
- 4 corn tortillas, gluten-free
- ¼ cup fresh cilantro, chopped
- 1 can (15 oz) black beans, drained and rinsed
- 2 ripe avocados
- 1 cup cherry tomatoes, diced
- ⅛ tsp salt
- ¼ cup red onion, finely chopped
- ⅛ tsp pepper

Directions:

1. In a bowl, mash the ripe avocados and add the lime juice, salt, and pepper. Mix well to create guacamole.
2. Warm the corn tortillas in a dry skillet or microwave.
3. Spread the guacamole onto each tortilla.
4. Top with black beans, cherry tomatoes, red onion, and fresh cilantro.
5. Serve as tacos or fold them into a burrito.

Special notes:

With a dash of hot sauce or jalapeños for an extra kick, you can spoil yourself while getting plenty of fiber, plant-based protein, and some healthy fats!

Salmon and Asparagus With Lemon Dill Sauce

A high-protein, low-carb option rich in omega-3 fatty acids.

Time: 19 minutes

Servings: 2

Nutritional information:

Calories	165
Carbs	8.8 grams
Protein	5 grams
Fat	14.3 grams

Ingredients:

- ¼ tsp oregano
- 4 salmon filets (6 oz each)
- 1 lemon, sliced
- ⅛ tsp pepper
- 2 tbsp olive oil
- 1 lb asparagus spears
- ⅛ tsp salt

Directions:

1. Drizzle the salmon filets with olive oil, sprinkle some oregano, and follow up with some salt and pepper.
2. Set your oven temperature to 400°F (200°C), then place the seasoned salmon on a baking sheet.
3. On top of each filet, place the lemon slices, then surround the salmon with asparagus. Drizzle the asparagus with some oil, sprinkle the pepper, oregano, and salt.

4. Roast for 13 to 17 minutes. When the salmon easily flakes with a fork, remove from the oven and serve.

Special notes:

You can use a light lemon dill sauce when serving this low-carb option for post-fasting meals. The dish is rich in omega-3 fatty acids, which are excellent for brain and heart health.

Mediterranean Chickpea Salad

This is a refreshing and protein-packed salad with a Mediterranean twist.

Time: 4

Servings: 2

Nutritional Information:

Calories	631
Carbs	76.3 grams
Protein	24.6 grams
Fat	28.1 grams

Ingredients:

- ¼ cup fresh parsley, chopped
- (15 oz each) chickpeas, drained and rinsed

- 2 tbsp red wine vinegar
- ½ cup red onion, finely chopped
- 1 cucumber, diced
- ⅛ tsp pepper
- ¼ cup crumbled feta cheese
- 2 tbsp extra virgin olive oil
- 1 tsp dried oregano
- 1 cup cherry tomatoes, halved
- ⅛ tsp salt
- ½ cup Kalamata olives, pitted and sliced

Directions:

1. For the salad, prepare a large bowl, then bring together the Kalamata olives, cucumber, chickpeas, red onion, fresh parsley, and cherry tomatoes.
2. If you're adding feta cheese, gently fold it into the salad, then prepare a separate small bowl.
3. Put the salt, dried oregano, and pepper into the second bowl, then whisk the red wine vinegar and olive oil in to make your dressing.
4. Drizzle the dressing over your chickpea salad and mix it in, then leave it to meld the flavors.
5. Serve the salad and enjoy.

Special notes:

You can improve this salad by adding grilled chicken or shrimp for extra protein. It's a great choice for a vegetarian or vegan post-fast meal.

Spiced Sweet Potato and Lentil Soup

This hearty soup is an excellent source of fiber and complex carbohydrates.

Time: 27 minutes

Servings: 2

Nutritional information:

Calories	345
Carbs	41.8 grams
Protein	18.4 grams
Fat	11.6 grams

Ingredients:

- ⅛ tsp pepper
- 6 cups vegetable broth
- 1 tsp ground cumin
- 1 onion, chopped
- 2 large sweet potatoes, peeled and diced
- 2 cloves garlic, minced
- 1 tbsp olive oil

- ½ tsp smoked paprika
- 1 cup green or brown lentils
- 1 tsp ground coriander
- ⅛ tsp salt

Directions:

1. Prepare a large pot over medium heat and pour the olive oil in. Throw the chopped onion in and sauté until translucent, then throw in the ground cumin and minced garlic.
2. Add the smoked paprika and ground coriander, and cook for another minute to release the flavors.
3. Mix the vegetable broth in, then add the lentils and sweet potatoes.
4. Bring the soup to a boil and reduce the heat, leaving it to simmer for about 23 minutes.
5. After the lentils and sweet potatoes become tender, puree the soup with an immersion blender, then season with salt and pepper.
6. Top with a dollop of Greek yogurt or garnish with fresh herbs.

Special notes:

This recipe is perfect for a warm, comforting post-fast meal.

Zucchini Noodles With Pesto

A low-carb, veggie-packed dish with zucchini noodles and a flavorful pesto sauce.

Time: 5 minutes

Servings: 2

Nutritional information:

Calories	628
Carbs	16.8 grams
Protein	8.8 grams
Fat	63.6 grams

Ingredients:

- 2 tbsp lemon juice
- ¼ cup grated Parmesan cheese
- 1 cup fresh basil leaves
- ⅛ tsp salt
- ½ cup extra virgin olive oil
- 4 medium zucchinis, spiralized into noodles
- ⅛ tsp pepper
- ¼ cup pine nuts
- 2 cloves garlic

Directions:

1. In a food processor, combine basil leaves, Parmesan cheese, pine nuts, and garlic.
2. Drizzle in some lemon juice and oil while pulsing the mixture. Continue blending until the pesto is smooth.
3. In a large pan, heat a bit of olive oil over medium heat, then cook the zucchini noodles for about 3 minutes.
4. When tender, mix the zucchini noodles with the freshly made pesto sauce until well-coated.
5. Season with salt and pepper to taste.

Special notes:

You can customize this dish by adding grilled shrimp, chicken, or tofu for extra protein. It's a low-carb, vegetarian option that's perfect for a light and satisfying post-fast meal.

Quinoa and Black Bean Salad

This high-protein and fiber-rich option suitable for vegetarians and vegans is another satisfying choice for a post-fast meal to keep you energized.

Time: 9 minutes

Servings: 2

Nutritional information:

Calories	864
Carbs	137.1 grams
Protein	36.6 grams
Fat	21.9 grams

Ingredients:

- ⅛ tsp pepper
- 1 cup quinoa, thoroughly rinsed
- 1 tsp ground cumin
- 1 can (15 oz) black beans, drained and rinsed
- ½ red onion, finely chopped
- 3 tbsp lime juice
- 1 red bell pepper, diced
- 2 tbsp olive oil
- ¼ cup fresh cilantro, chopped
- ⅛ tsp salt
- 1 cup corn kernels (fresh, canned, or frozen)

Directions:

1. Cook the quinoa according to package instructions, then leave it to cool.
2. Prepare a large bowl and mix the black beans, cooked quinoa, corn, red onion, fresh cilantro, and red bell pepper together.

3. For the dressing, mix the pepper, lime juice, and ground cumin in a small bowl. Whisk in some olive oil and salt, then dress the salad.
4. Mix well before covering and placing in the freezer for a few minutes to serve chilled.

Special notes:

These recipes offer a range of nutrient-rich options for your post-fast meals, catering to various dietary preferences and providing balanced nutrition to fuel your fasting body.

A PEEK INTO THE DIET TRACKER SHEET

A diet tracker sheet is a useful tool that can help you with intermittent fasting. It gives you a way to keep track of your meals and fasting times, making it easy to stay on track and make smart choices about your nutrition and eating routine. You can adjust this tracker to fit any intermittent fasting approach.

Its primary purposes include nutrition analysis, meal planning, and tracking fasting windows. Foods that are high in carbs, protein, and fat are clearly broken down in the sheet for each meal. This information is important for nutrition analysis because it helps you keep your food balanced and make any changes that are needed.

The sheet lets you plan your meals ahead of time, so you can make sure you eat a healthy diet during your eating times. You can keep track of your fasting periods to make sure you stick to the intermittent fasting plan you choose. The diet tracker also keeps track of how much water you drink, which is very important when you are fasting.

If you fill out your diet tracker sheet on a regular basis, you can learn more about what you eat and how it affects your energy, mood, and general health. This tool is great for your intermittent fasting journey as it gives you the information you need to make smart decisions and get the most out of intermittent fasting. Below is a sample diet tracker sheet you can use.

Day	Time	Food or Water Intake	Nutritional Information	Notes, Observations, or Reminders

CONCLUSION

Intermittent fasting is a powerful tool that empowers you to reclaim your health and prime years. Remember to also focus on when and how you nourish your body, rather than only worrying about what you eat. We've explored the science behind this eating approach, looked into some inspiring stories, and covered some practical strategies that can reshape your life.

Now, you have the power to unlock your potential for a healthier and happier life in and beyond your 50s. It's time to take the best next step and integrate these valuable insights into your daily life. Empower yourself to make every moment count, and remember: Your best years are yet to come!

I'd love to read about your thoughts and experiences with this book. If you found my advice helpful, please leave a review, and let's inspire other women to improve their lives too!

REFERENCES

Allen, L. H. (2012). Vitamin B-12. *Advances in Nutrition, 3*(1), 54–55. https://doi.org/10.3945/an.111.001370

Anagnostis, P., Lambrinoudaki, I., Stevenson, J. C., & Goulis, D. G. (2022). Menopause-associated risk of cardiovascular disease. *Endocrine Connections, 11*(4). https://doi.org/10.1530/EC-21-0537

Bass, A. D., Van Wijmeersch, B., Mayer, L., Mäurer, M., Boster, A., Mandel, M., Mitchell, C., Sharrock, K., & Singer, B. (2019). Effect of multiple sclerosis on daily activities, emotional well-being, and relationships. *International Journal of MS Care, 22*(4), 158–164. https://doi.org/10.7224/1537-2073.2018-087

Bedosky, L. (n.d.). *Low-impact workouts: What they are, health benefits, and getting started.* EverydayHealth.com. https://www.everydayhealth.com/fitness/low-impact-workouts/guide/

Berchtold, M. W., Brinkmeier, H., & Müntener, M. (2000). Calcium ion in skeletal muscle: Its crucial role for muscle function, plasticity, and disease. *Physiological Reviews, 80*(3), 1215–1265. https://doi.org/10.1152/physrev.2000.80.3.1215

Borchert, R., & McChesney, J. D. (1973). Time course and localization of DNA synthesis during wound healing of potato tuber tissue. *Developmental Biology, 35*(2), 293–301. https://doi.org/10.1016/0012-1606(73)90025-0

Brody, B. (n.d.). *11 easy ways to get more water.* WebMD; WebMD. Retrieved January 17, 2020, from https://www.webmd.com/diet/drink-more-water-tips

Brown, E. (n.d.). *How to qualify for social security benefits with osteoporosis.* Verywell Health. Retrieved October 23, 2023, from https://www.verywellhealth.com/is-osteoporosis-a-disability-6827097

Carr, A. J., Gibson, B., & Robinson, P. G. (2001). Is quality of life determined by expectations or experience? *BMJ : British Medical Journal, 322*(7296), 1240–1243. https://www.ncbi.nlm.nih.gov/pmc/articles/PMC1120338/

CDC. (2022, January 5). *Physical activity for arthritis | CDC.* Www.cdc.gov. https://www.cdc.gov/arthritis/basics/physical-activity/index.html

Centers for Disease Control and Prevention. (2018, June 12). *Attempts to lose weight among adults in the United States, 2013–2016.* CDC. https://www.cdc.gov/nchs/products/databriefs/db313.htm

Chan, K. (n.d.). *Empty nest syndrome: How to cope when the kids flee the coop.* Verywell Mind. Retrieved October 23, 2023, from https://www.verywellmind.com/empty-nest-syndrome-how-to-cope-when-the-kids-flee-the-coop-7480061

Collins, R. (2012, March 29). *Exercise, depression, and the brain.* Healthline; Healthline Media. https://www.healthline.com/health/depression/exercise

Coulter, A., & Oldham, J. (2016). Person-centred care: What is it and how do we get there? *Future Hospital Journal, 3*(2), 114–116. https://www.ncbi.nlm.nih.gov/pmc/articles/PMC6465833/

De Rechter, S., Decuypere, J.-P., Ivanova, E., van den Heuvel, L. P., De Smedt, H., Levtchenko, E., & Mekahli, D. (2015). Autophagy in renal diseases. *Pediatric Nephrology, 31*(5), 737–752. https://doi.org/10.1007/s00467-015-3134-2

Dhurandhar, E. J., Dawson, J., Alcorn, A., Larsen, L. H., Thomas, E. A., Cardel, M., Bourland, A. C., Astrup, A., St-Onge, M.-P., Hill, J. O., Apovian, C. M., Shikany, J. M., & Allison, D. B. (2014). The effectiveness of breakfast recommendations on weight loss: a randomized controlled trial. *The American Journal of Clinical Nutrition, 100*(2), 507–513. https://doi.org/10.3945/ajcn.114.089573

Evolve MMA. (n.d.). 6 types of intermittent fasting schedules that produce results. *Evolve Daily.* https://evolve-mma.com/blog/6-types-of-intermittent-fasting-schedules-that-produce-results/

Fletcher, J. (2019, December 16). *The best time to take vitamins: Recommendations for different types.* Www.medicalnewstoday.com. https://www.medicalnewstoday.com/articles/319556

Getsmarter. (2020, February 14). *What are macronutrients and micronutrients.* GetSmarter Blog. https://www.getsmarter.com/blog/market-trends/what-are-macronutrients-and-micronutrients/

Gîlcă, M., Soian, I., Mohora, M., Petec, C., Muscurel, C., & Dinu, V. (2003). The effect of fasting on the parameters of the antioxidant defence system in the blood of vegetarian human subjects. *Romanian Journal of Internal Medicine = Revue Roumaine de Medecine Interne*, *41*(3), 283–292. https://pubmed.ncbi.nlm.nih.gov/15526512/

Gill, L. E., Bartels, S. J., & Batsis, J. A. (2015). Weight management in older adults. *Current Obesity Reports*, *4*(3), 379–388. https://doi.org/10.1007/s13679-015-0161-z

Grant, M. D., Marbella, A., Wang, A. T., Pines, E., Hoag, J., Bonnell, C., Ziegler, K. M., & Aronson, N. (2015). Introduction. In *www.ncbi.nlm.nih.gov*. Agency for Healthcare Research and Quality (US). https://www.ncbi.nlm.nih.gov/books/NBK285446/

Harvard T.H. Chan. (2012, October 21). *Health risks*. Obesity Prevention Source. https://www.hsph.harvard.edu/obesity-prevention-source/obesity-consequences/health-effects/

Hever, J., & Cronise, R. J. (2017). Plant-based nutrition for healthcare professionals: Implementing diet as a primary modality in the prevention and treatment of chronic disease. *Journal of Geriatric Cardiology : JGC*, *14*(5), 355–368. https://doi.org/10.11909/j.issn.1671-5411.2017.05.012

Hiller-Sturmhöfel, S., & Bartke, A. (1998). The endocrine system: An overview. *Alcohol Health and Research World*, *22*(3), 153–164. https://www.ncbi.nlm.nih.gov/pmc/articles/PMC6761896/

Huskisson, E., Maggini, S., & Ruf, M. (2007). The role of vitamins and minerals in energy metabolism and well-being. *Journal of International Medical Research*, *35*(3), 277–289. https://doi.org/10.1177/147323000703500301

Jeanine, & Jack. (n.d.). *Greek salad dressing*. Love and Lemons. https://www.loveandlemons.com/greek-salad-dressing/

Kameda, T., Mano, H., Yuasa, T., Mori, Y., Miyazawa, K., Shiokawa, M., Nakamaru, Y., Hiroi, E., Hiura, K., Kameda, A., Yang, N. N., Hakeda, Y., & Kumegawa, M. (1997). Estrogen inhibits bone resorption by directly inducing apoptosis of the bone-resorbing osteoclasts. *The Journal of Experimental Medicine*, *186*(4), 489–495. https://www.ncbi.nlm.nih.gov/pmc/articles/PMC2199029/

Kandola, A. (2023, April 17). *Top 5 intermittent fasting benefits ranked.* https://www.medicalnewstoday.com/articles/323605

Katz, D. L., Doughty, K., & Ali, A. (2011). Cocoa and chocolate in human health and disease. *Antioxidants & Redox Signaling, 15*(10), 2779–2811. https://doi.org/10.1089/ars.2010.3697

Kim, J. Y. (2020). Optimal diet strategies for weight loss and weight loss maintenance. *Journal of Obesity & Metabolic Syndrome, 30*(1). https://doi.org/10.7570/jomes20065

Leonard, J. (n.d.). *7 ways to do intermittent fasting: Best methods and quick tips.* Medical News Today. https://www.medicalnewstoday.com/articles/322293

Manami. (n.d.). *Brown rice stir-fry with flavored tofu and vegetables recipe.* https://www.food.com/recipe/brown-rice-stir-fry-with-flavored-tofu-and-vegetables-207869

Manoogian, E. N. C., & Laferrère, B. (2023). Time-restricted eating: What we know and where the field is going. *Obesity, 31*(S1), 7–8. https://doi.org/10.1002/oby.23672

Mark, C. (2022, October 13). *52% of the world's adults are trying to lose weight. Who are they?* Business.yougov.com. https://business.yougov.com/content/44057-52-worlds-adults-trying-lose-weight

Mcmurray, R. G., Soares, J., Caspersen, C. J., & Mccurdy, T. (2014). Examining variations of resting metabolic rate of adults. *Medicine & Science in Sports & Exercise, 46*(7), 1352–1358. https://doi.org/10.1249/mss.0000000000000232

MGH Center for Women's Mental Health. (2017, February 1). *In brief: Why exercise helps with menopausal hot flashes.* https://womensmentalhealth.org/posts/brief-exercise-helps-menopausal-hot-flashes/

Miller, V. M., Kling, J. M., Files, J. A., Joyner, M. J., Kapoor, E., Moyer, A. M., Rocca, W. A., & Faubion, S. S. (2018). What's in a name: Are menopausal "hot flashes" a symptom of menopause or a manifestation of neurovascular dysregulation?. *Menopause, 25*(6), 700–703. https://doi.org/10.1097/gme.0000000000001065

Mongraw-Chaffin, M., Beavers, D. P., & McClainc, D. A. (2019). Hypoglycemic symptoms in the absence of diabetes: Pilot evidence of clinical hypoglycemia in young women. *Journal of Clinical &*

Translational Endocrinology, 18, 100202. https://doi.org/10.1016/j.jcte.2019.100202

Morin, A. (2019). *5 signs and symptoms of empty nest syndrome*. Verywell Family. https://www.verywellfamily.com/signs-of-empty-nest-syndrome-4163787

Mulas, A., Cienfuegos, S., Ezpeleta, M., Lin, S., Pavlou, V., & Varady, K. A. (2023). Effect of intermittent fasting on circulating inflammatory markers in obesity: A review of human trials. *Frontiers in Nutrition, 10*. https://doi.org/10.3389/fnut.2023.1146924

Nall, R. (2019, February 22). *How do I determine the macronutrient content of fresh foods?* Healthline. https://healthline.com/nutrition/macronutrient-info-for-unlabeled-foods#5

National Cancer Institute. (2020, February 18). *Physical activity and cancer fact sheet*. https://www.cancer.gov/about-cancer/causes-prevention/risk/obesity/physical-activity-fact-sheet

National Institute of Health. (2022, September 27). *Vitamin D for heart health: Where the benefits begin and end*. Www.nhlbi.nih.gov. https://www.nhlbi.nih.gov/news/2022/vitamin-d-heart-health-where-benefits-begin-and-end

National Institute on Aging. (n.d.). *Healthy meal planning: Tips for older adults*. National Institute on Aging. https://www.nia.nih.gov/health/healthy-meal-planning-tips-older-adults

Osilla, E. V., Safadi, A. O., & Sharma, S. (2020). *Calories*. PubMed; StatPearls Publishing. https://www.ncbi.nlm.nih.gov/books/NBK499909/

Panuganti, K. K., Nguyen, M., & Kshirsagar, R. K. (2022). *Obesity*. PubMed; StatPearls Publishing. https://www.ncbi.nlm.nih.gov/books/NBK459357/

Patterson, R. E., Laughlin, G. A., LaCroix, A. Z., Hartman, S. J., Natarajan, L., Senger, C. M., Martínez, M. E., Villaseñor, A., Sears, D. D., Marinac, C. R., & Gallo, L. C. (2015). Intermittent fasting and human metabolic health. *Journal of the Academy of Nutrition and Dietetics, 115*(8), 1203–1212. https://doi.org/10.1016/j.jand.2015.02.018

PBS Food. (n.d.). *Caesar salad tacos recipe*. PBS Food. Retrieved October

23, 2023, from https://www.pbs.org/food/recipes/caesar-salad-tacos/

Schorr, M., Dichtel, L. E., Gerweck, A. V., Valera, R. D., Torriani, M., Miller, K. K., & Bredella, M. A. (2018). Sex differences in body composition and association with cardiometabolic risk. *Biology of Sex Differences*, *9*(1). https://doi.org/10.1186/s13293-018-0189-3

Song, C., Yao, L., Chen, H., Song, Y., & Liu, L. (2023). Prevalence and factors influencing depression among empty nesters in China: A meta-analysis. *BMC Geriatrics*, *23*, 333. https://doi.org/10.1186/s12877-023-04064-0

Stipp, D. (2013, January 1). *How intermittent fasting might help you live a longer and healthier life*. Scientific American. https://www.scientificamerican.com/article/how-intermittent-fasting-might-help-you-live-longer-healthier-life/

Thielke, S., Sale, J., & Reid, M. C. (2012). Aging: Are these 4 pain myths complicating care? *The Journal of Family Practice*, *61*(11), 666–670. https://www.ncbi.nlm.nih.gov/pmc/articles/PMC4356472/

Thurrott, S. (2022, September 20). *How retirement afforded 1 woman the time to walk off 90 pounds*. TODAY.com. https://www.today.com/health/diet-fitness/90-pound-weight-loss-walking-intermittent-fasting-rcna47388

USDA. (2015). *Dietary guidelines for Americans eighth edition*. https://health.gov/sites/default/files/2019-09/2015-2020_Dietary_Guidelines.pdf

Vasim, I., Majeed, C. N., & DeBoer, M. D. (2022). Intermittent fasting and metabolic health. *Nutrients*, *14*(3), 631. https://doi.org/10.3390/nu14030631

Vieira, A. F., Costa, R. R., Macedo, R. C. O., Coconcelli, L., & Kruel, L. F. M. (2016). Effects of aerobic exercise performed in fasted v. fed state on fat and carbohydrate metabolism in adults: a systematic review and meta-analysis. *British Journal of Nutrition*, *116*(7), 1153–1164. https://doi.org/10.1017/s0007114516003160

Visioli, F., Mucignat-Caretta, C., Anile, F., & Panaite, S.-A. (2022). Traditional and medical applications of fasting. *Nutrients*, *14*(3), 433. https://doi.org/10.3390/nu14030433

Volpi, E., Nazemi, R., & Fujita, S. (2004). Muscle tissue changes with aging. *Current Opinion in Clinical Nutrition and Metabolic Care, 7*(4), 405–410. https://www.ncbi.nlm.nih.gov/pmc/articles/PMC2804956/

Waehner, P. (n.d.). *How many calories does muscle really burn?* Verywell Fit. https://www.verywellfit.com/how-many-calories-does-muscle-really-burn-1231074

Watkins, E., & Serpell, L. (2016). The psychological effects of short-term fasting in healthy women. *Frontiers in Nutrition, 3.* https://doi.org/10.3389/fnut.2016.00027

Welton, S., Minty, R., O'Driscoll, T., Willms, H., Poirier, D., Madden, S., & Kelly, L. (2020). Intermittent fasting and weight loss. *Canadian Family Physician, 66*(2), 117–125. https://www.ncbi.nlm.nih.gov/pmc/articles/PMC7021351/

Westcott, W. L. (2012). Resistance training is medicine: Effects of strength training on health. *Current Sports Medicine Reports, 11*(4), 209–216. https://doi.org/10.1249/JSR.0b013e31825dabb8

Wicherski, J., Schlesinger, S., & Fischer, F. (2021). Association between breakfast skipping and body weight—a systematic review and meta-analysis of observational longitudinal studies. *Nutrients, 13*(1), 272. https://doi.org/10.3390/nu13010272

Wilhelmi de Toledo, F., Grundler, F., Bergouignan, A., Drinda, S., & Michalsen, A. (2019). Safety, health improvement and well-being during a 4 to 21-day fasting period in an observational study including 1422 subjects. *PLOS ONE, 14*(1), e0209353. https://doi.org/10.1371/journal.pone.0209353

Wooll, M. (2022, January 13). *Empty nest syndrome: How to cope when kids fly the coop.* https://www.betterup.com/blog/empty-nest-syndrome

Yao, Ding, Wang, Jin, Lin, Zhai, Zhang, He, & Fan. (2019). Risk factors for depression in empty nesters: A cross-sectional study in a coastal city of Zhejiang province and china. *International Journal of Environmental Research and Public Health, 16*(21), 4106. https://doi.org/10.3390/ijerph16214106

Zehnacker, C. H., & Bemis-Dougherty, A. (2007). Effect of weighted exercises on bone mineral density in post menopausal women a systematic review. *Journal of Geriatric Physical Therapy, 30*(2), 79–88. https://doi.org/10.1519/00139143-200708000-00007

Acknowledgments

I wish to express my sincere gratitude to Samaria, without whom this book would be nothing more than a dream!

Printed in Great Britain
by Amazon

39012274R00118